# HAND
# INJURIES

# HAND INJURIES
## A THERAPEUTIC APPROACH

**MAUREEN I. SALTER** MBE MCSP

Formerly Superintendent Physiotherapist, RAF Chessington, Surrey

*With contributions by*

**Alison T. Davis** MCSP

Formerly Senior Physiotherapist, The Regional Burns and Plastic Surgery Unit,
Queen Mary's Hospital, Roehampton

**Heather Unsworth** DipCOT SETC

Research and Training Occupational Therapist, Odstock Hospital, Salisbury

*Foreword by*

**C.B. Wynn Parry** MBE DM FRCP FRCS

Director of Rehabilitation, Royal National Orthopaedic Hospital, Stanmore, Middlesex

**Churchill Livingstone**

EDINBURGH LONDON MELBOURNE AND NEW YORK 1987

CHURCHILL LIVINGSTONE
Medical Division of Longman Group UK Limited

Distributed in the United States of America by Churchill
Livingstone Inc., 1560 Broadway, New York, N.Y. 10036,
and by associated companies, branches and representatives
throughout the world.

First published 1987

ISBN  0-443-02984-9

British Library Cataloguing in Publication Data
Salter, Maureen
    Hand injuries.
    1. Hand—Wounds and injuries—Treatment
    2. Physical therapy
    I. Title
    617'.575044     RC951

Library of Congress Cataloging in Publication Data
Salter, Maureen I.
    Hand injuries.
    Includes index.
    1. Hand—Wounds and injuries—Treatment. I. Davis,
Alison T. II. Title. [DNLM: 1. Hand Injuries—therapy.
WE 830 S177h]
    RD559.S24     1987     617'.575044     87-756

Produced by Longman Singapore Publishers (Pte) Ltd.
Printed in Singapore

# Foreword

It is a pleasure to introduce this book specifically designed for hand therapists by one of the leading hand physiotherapists in Britain.

Maureen Salter set a standard of assessment and management of complex hand disabilities at the RAF Rehabilitation Centre at Chessington that has never been surpassed.

Her attention to detail, insistence on intensive and frequent treatment sessions, her careful records and skilled manual techniques helped countless servicemen to return to duty despite severe injury.

Just as important has been her dedication to teaching and the selfless way she has taken on generations of students who have carried her message far and wide.

She has always recognised the importance of the team in rehabilitation and so this book pays tribute to the vital role of the occupational therapist, as well as the psychologist, nurse and gymnast.

This manual will appeal to all members of the hand service, doctors as well as therapists. It is a fitting climax to a brilliant career.

C.B.W.P.

# Preface

Repeated suggestions from fellow physiotherapists plus some prompting from the editors at Churchill Livingstone finally persuaded me to write this book. It is aimed primarily for physiotherapists, either those who are newly entering the exciting field of specialised hand management or those who treat few rather than many hand injuries. Hopefully it may be of interest to occupational therapists also. Although the majority of hand injuries are non-problematical it is inevitable that a proportion become complicated. An attempt is made to explain the complexities and assist the therapist in both assessing the problems and deciding the priorities of treatment.

An appointment as a physiotherapist at RAF Chessington twenty five years ago first introduced me to the rehabilitation of hands, and my interest has remained unfailing ever since. Without this experience at Chessington this book could never have been contemplated.

A particular privilege was to have worked for many of those years with Dr Kit Wynn Parry. Not only myself but many others have benefited from his vast knowledge of hands and his willingness to impart this information. I am especially grateful to him for reading the manuscript and for making some valuable comments. Some of the work described in this book was developed during those years at Chessington and is already in print in Dr Wynn Parry's book *Rehabilitation of the Hand*, published by Butterworths.

My sincere thanks go to my colleagues for their contributions to this book: Alison Davies for her chapter on the burnt hand, and Heather Unsworth for both the chapter on occupational therapy and for the sections on the power, functional and work assessments, the Odstock measurements and for the discussion on the psychological aspects of hand injuries. This book would not be complete without their excellent contributions on these specialised subjects.

I should like to acknowledge all that I have learnt over the years from so many other colleagues, both doctors and therapists, with whom I have worked. To include everyone would take too long but I would especially like to mention physiotherapists Barbara Sutcliffe, Oona Scott, Jane Stichbury and Freda Lewis, and occupational therapists Natalie Barr and Doris Millar. Recently I have had tremendous support in my project from Joy Hill, Julie Evans, Nigel Hanchard and other colleagues at Chessington both serving and civilian. My thanks go also to Susan Boardman of Mount Vernon for support and encouragement and for the provision of photographs for Figures 3.57 and 4.2a Membership of the physiotherapist's hand discussion group has also provided a source of knowledge, interest and stimulation since its conception several years ago.

My particular thanks go to Norman Chandler of the Medical Photography Department at RAF Halton for the photographs, whose excellent quality is evident throughout this book. His advice and the standard of his photography at Chessington for more than twenty years has been highly valued. I wish also to acknowledge the kind permission of the Director General of Medical Services, Royal Air Force to publish this book.

The assistance and advice of editors and staff at Churchill Livingstone have been of great help to me. They have been most patient with my problems and the length of time it has taken me to finish the book.

Lastly I am grateful to my husband and friends for their continued support and understanding whilst I struggled with the manuscript. In particular I should like to mention my friend Katie Hooker. Without her constant help and her assistance with the typing this book could never have been completed.

Sadly RAF Chessington is no longer a rehabilitation unit, but its work continues at RAF Headley Court. I should like to dedicate this book to all the staff and patients who, during its forty years existence, made Chessington such a memorable unit.

West Sussex, 1987                                        M.S.

# Contents

# 1

# Function of the hand

Man is capable of achieving a wide variety of functions and skills with his hand, and the learning process commences at a very early age. During his first six weeks, when grasping a finger or an object placed in his hand, the baby is not only utilising reflex activity, but also gaining knowledge from the novel sensory input. As his voluntary movements increase the child will learn, by feeling objects and by using all the other sensory modalities such as watching, listening and testing in his mouth. These stimuli help him to ratify his cutaneous sensibility without which he could not build his repertoire of motor activity.

An early achievement is to roll over into the prone position when he will learn to extend his fingers and support himself on his forearms, thus acquiring stability of his trunk on his hands. This is influenced by the sensory input from the skin and the proprioception of his joints.

At four and a half months he is starting to reach out independently for toys and to co-ordinate his movements. During the following months he will acquire the skill of prehension, gradually improving the stability of his upper arm and the co-ordination of his hand (Horton 1971).

Encouragement and help from his mother are vital for the normal development of the child. A large part of his early life is occupied at play, and much of this time will be spent using his hands for his activities. Children who are deprived of these opportunities are likely to be psychologically affected for the rest of their lives.

Evolution over many generations has produced variations from the squat, muscular hand of the

1

labourer to the long tapering fingers and mobile hand of the dancer and artist. It is these latter mobile hands which are more vulnerable to severe injury and take longer to rehabilitate.

## FUNCTIONS

The main functions of the hand, and those which need to be restored following injury are:

1. Grasp
2. Support
3. Striking movements
4. Free movements
5. Communication and expression
6. Sensory organ
7. Orientation.

### GRASP

The variations of grip, or prehension, are adjustable according to the size, shape and solidity of the object to be held. Sufficient finger extension must also be available for first grasping and then releasing the object.

### (i) Power grip

The fingers and thumb are flexed around the object with the wrist stabilised in slight extension. The power in this grip is mainly provided by the strength of the ring and little finger opposing that of the thumb. The object lies diagonally across the palm, with the metacarpophalangeal joints in ulnar deviation and slight rotation to maintain strong finger contact.

Power grip may be double-handed for activities needing great strength and stability such as using a shovel or pick-axe when the whole arm moves and the long flexors of the fingers contract strongly to maintain the grasp (Fig. 1.1). Power grip may also be single-handed, as in holding a hammer, the thumb lying on the shaft directing the hammer head while the movement takes place at the wrist.

An adaptation of this grip is to add some precision, e.g. holding a knife and fork. The implements are held firmly by the ring and little fingers with the index fingers guiding the line of movement. The full flexion of the little and ring

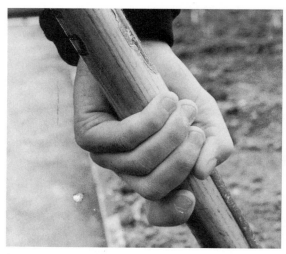

**Fig. 1.1** Strong grasp. Note power of thumb opposing little and ring fingers, with less strength of index and middle fingers.

fingers into the palm prevents a screwdriver from sliding through the hand when pressure is applied.

### (ii) Precision grip

This is the most frequently used form of grasp. Accurate and precise movements can be achieved by application of the tips of fingers and thumb, utilising the skin areas with maximum sensory supply. The extent of finger area used will depend on the weight or delicacy of the object being picked up, and on the task to be undertaken.

a. *Pinch or lateral grip*, e.g. holding a key whilst inserting it into a lock (Fig. 1.2): this entails

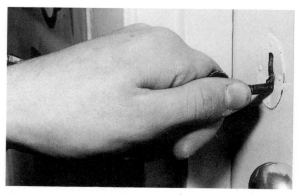

**Fig. 1.2** Lateral pinch grip. Note activity of 1st dorsal interosseous.

opposition of the palmar surface of the thumb tip against the lateral surface of the index distal phalanx. There is a strong contraction of the first dorsal interosseous and adductor pollicis, stabilised with lateral support from the middle finger.

Interdigital pinch is utilised by the smoker when holding a cigarette between index and middle fingers.

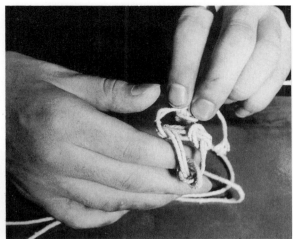

**Fig. 1.4** Use of the nails to unpick string.

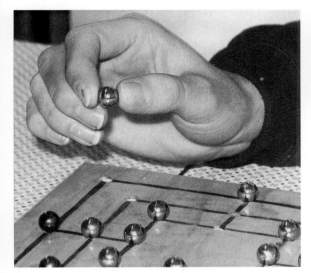

**Fig. 1.3** Tip grip using finger and thumb only: the smaller the object the greater degree of joint flexion that is required.

b. *Tip grip* is used for small and delicate objects (Fig. 1.3). It may utilise index finger and thumb only, or the thumb with two or three fingers, depending on the diameter of the object.

The nails can be used to pick up minute objects, to unpick knots (Fig. 1.4), and to scrape the surface such as removing a sticky label off a jar or adhesive tape from the skin. The skin of the finger tips is used for leafing through papers and bank notes. The slight degree of normal skin sweating makes adherence possible.

Awareness of skin and nail use is enhanced by the excellent sensory nerve supply of digit tips and nail beds and particularly of the dynamic sides of the thumb and index finger.

c. *Span grip* involves all the fingers, and the five digit tips are able to encircle the object due to the arch structure of the hand (Fig. 1.5a). Contact with more of the finger surface may be required when a slightly heavier object is grasped (Fig. 1.5b).

d. *Tripod grip*, with the palmar surfaces of the distal phalanges of thumb and index finger rotated towards one another, is supported laterally by the middle finger. Delicate support of paintbrush pen and pencil are examples (Figs. 1.6a & b).

### (iii) Hook grip

With the fingers flexed strongly at the proximal interphalangeal joints the endurance power of flexor digitorum superficialis is utilised. It is demonstrated when objects such as a bucket or suitcase are carried, and the contraction, mainly of flexor digitorum superficialis, has the effect of flattening the arches (Fig. 1.7).

### SUPPORT

Body weight may be supported on the hand:
(i) Total hand support, which is a primitive use, should be regained as soon as possible following injury. The child has learnt the action early when crawling and later when performing hand-stands and cart-wheels. While leaning on the whole hand we can support and balance ourselves by stabilising the trunk on the arm.
(ii) Thumb and finger tips steady paper or position a ruler whilst a pen or pencil is used with the other hand (Fig. 1.8).

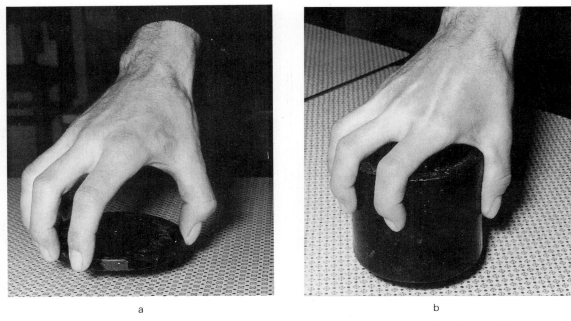

**Fig. 1.5** Span grip: (a) using the tips of the digits for a light weight. (b) using a greater surface for a heavier object. Note altered position of metacarpophalangeal joints.

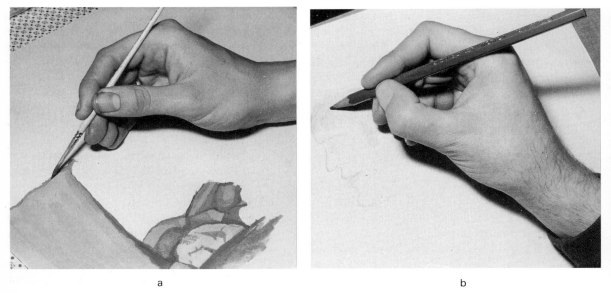

**Fig. 1.6** Dynamic tripod grip: (a) for delicate touch. (b) for firmer pressure. Note the altered positions of the joints and also the support given by the little finger.

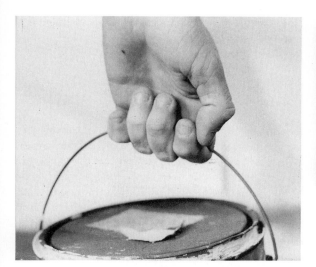

**Fig. 1.7** Hook grip. Note the flattening of the arches and also that the majority of finger flexion is at the proximal interphalangeal joints.

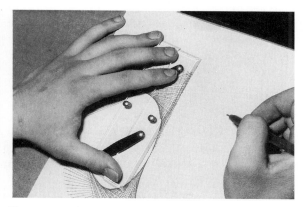

**Fig. 1.8** Steadying support using finger tips.

(iii) Little finger support allows skilled activities to be carried out by thumb, index and middle fingers, e.g. when writing. The hand can be positioned correctly because of the isometric contraction of the abductor digiti minimi and other hypothenar muscles. The amputation of a little finger can therefore be a very disabling injury.

## STRIKING MOVEMENTS

These movements are accomplished with fingers totally flexed as for a punch (Fig. 1.9) or extended

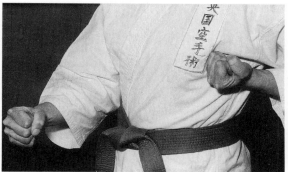

**Fig. 1.9** Striking power.

as for karate. The hand, utilising the strength of the whole arm, can be a powerful weapon for both aggression and protection.

## FREE MOVEMENTS

Simple movements of stroking, caressing and wiping utilise the activity of the whole arm with a statically positioned hand.

Fast intricate movement of the fingers, as when typing and playing musical instruments, requires each hand to be independent of the other (Fig. 1.10). This is possible only when there is stability of the upper arm. A large degree of movement occurs at the metacarpophalangeal joints, and is monitored closely by feedback from the lumbrical muscles in particular. These movements, which are highly skilled, develop during childhood and are dependent on good sensibility of the hand.

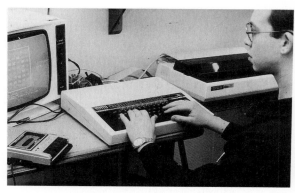

**Fig. 1.10** Free skilled movements, the fingers of each hand moving individually.

## COMMUNICATION AND EXPRESSION

A variety of gestures is used for communication, from simple greetings to the complex sign language of the deaf and dumb (Fig. 1.11). Gestures may be conscious or unconscious, and can denote love and respect or defiance and pure aggression. Dancers of many nations use their hands as a form of cultural expression. Their use is an integral but individual part of everyone's personality.

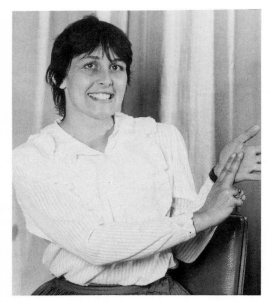

**Fig. 1.11**   Communication by sign language.

## SENSORY ORGAN

Sensibility of the hand is the means by which cutaneous and proprioceptive stimuli are utilised:
 (i) For achieving skilled motor function
 (ii) As a protection from injury, for awareness of touch and for testing temperature etc.
(iii) For recognition of objects by stereognosis.
 Sensory awareness, which we take for granted in our own lives, is absolutely essential for normal hand function. It is mostly combined with movement, so by this means can be influenced best after nerve injury. When a patient is specifically trained, a remarkable degree of awareness can be achieved, e.g. a blind person can learn to read Braille. If sen-sation does not recover adequately following a median nerve lesion the patient is less likely to use his hand efficiently.

## PERFORMANCE OF FUNCTIONAL MOVEMENT

In order to execute this wide variety of movements certain anatomical and physiological factors must be present. These include stability of the trunk and upper arm, which is necessary for the hand to be able to function at all, and both mobility and stability of the structures of the hand itself. The hand must be able to change rapidly from a flat support to a dynamic arch, in which position it performs most of its numerous roles.
 In the following pages some anatomical aspects affecting functional performance are mentioned which are of particular relevance to therapists. Detailed anatomy of bones, joints and ligaments, muscles, nerves and vascular supply can be found in the relevant anatomy textbooks, and in the numerous articles written by hand specialists (see References and Further Reading).

## ARCHES

The arches play an important role during activity as it is their adaptability which enables the hand to adjust to such a variety of situations. The main arches are:
1. Longitudinal
2. Transverse
3. Oblique.

### Longitudinal arch

This extends from the proximal row of the carpal bones to the tips of the fingers and thumb (Fig. 1.12). It is maintained largely by the tension between the long flexors and extensors of fingers and thumbs, with interaction of the intrinsic muscles.

### Transverse arches

These are found proximally through the carpal bones, and distally through the heads of the meta-carpals (Fig. 1.12). The effect continues to the tips

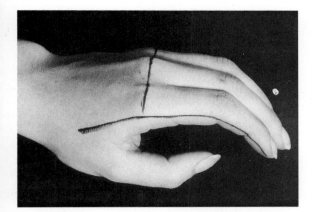

**Fig. 1.12**   The transverse and longitudinal arches.

of fingers and thumb, which remain in an arched position even when the hand is relaxed.

These transverse arches are maintained by the action of all the small muscles of the hand and their paralysis produces an arch collapse with resulting deformity and disability.

## Oblique arches

These arise from the thumb, when it is positioned in some degree of abduction and opposition, and extend into either the index or little finger

(Figs. 1.13a & b). They are maintained largely by the activity of thenar and hypothenar muscles. The fingers abduct automatically when they extend (Fig. 1.14a) and the transverse arch structure causes the tips to converge towards one another when they flex (Fig. 1.14b). This enables a firm grasp to be made around an object (Fig. 1.15). The index finger has the additional ability of rotation either towards the palm or towards the tip of the thumb (Figs. 1.16a & b).

The normal hand in repose assumes a position with the arches still present (Fig. 1.17). The wrist is usually slightly dorsiflexed: the metacarpophalangeal joints are flexed at about 25°, the proximal interphalangeal joints at 45° and the distal interphalangeal joints at about 15°. The thumb lies anterior to the second metacarpal and phalanges of the index finger. This is very similar to the *position of function* of the hand.

Visco-elastic tension, or tone, of the long flexors of fingers and thumb is slightly stronger than that of the extensors, thus a certain degree of finger flexion is maintained.

Any alteration from this normal position of rest is important to note when assessing disorders following injury. When exercising and splinting the hand it is essential that all arches should be maintained, especially when the intrinsic muscles are paralysed.

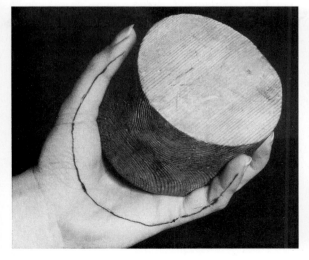

a

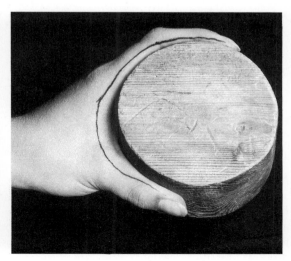

b

**Fig. 1.13(a & b)**   The oblique arches

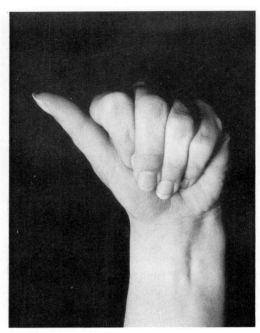

**Fig. 1.14** (a) The fingers abduct in extension (b) The tips converge in flexion.

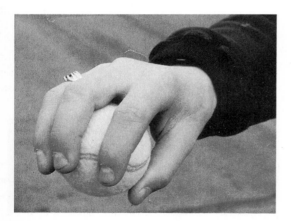

**Fig. 1.15** The arch formations allow a firm grasp to be made around the object.

## JOINTS

Both the shape of the joint surfaces and the position in which the ligaments lie are responsible for the direction and degree of movement that takes place at that joint. Synovial joints are classified as either ovoid or sellar (Williams & Warwick 1980).

1. *Ovoid*. In these articulations the convex male surface is larger than the female concave surface. There is considerable variation in shape, from being nearly flat to being nearly a sphere. They include the previous joint classifications: ball and socket (shoulder), plane (intercarpal), hinge (interphalangeal), ellipsoid (radio-carpal and metacarpophalangeal), and pivot (radio-ulnar) joints.

2. *Sellar*. Various planes of movement can occur at this joint, an example of this being the saddle joint of the carpometacarpal joint of the thumb.

### Movements

The movements which take place at the synovial joints are termed as either spin or swing.

1. Spin occurs at the shoulder and radio-humeral joints of the arm and also at the hip joint.

2. Swing occurs at all other joints. As joint surfaces are not totally congruent the swing component is made up of roll and slide movements. Some degree of rotation takes place at the majority of joints, and as this cannot be produced voluntarily it is termed *conjunct rotation*. MacConnaill (1964)

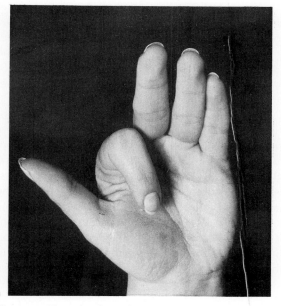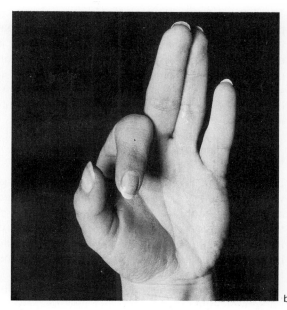

a  b

**Fig. 1.16**  The index finger flexing: (a) towards the palm (b) towards the thumb.

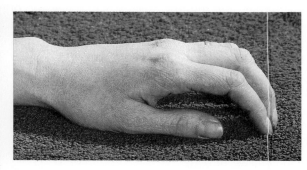

**Fig. 1.17**  The hand in repose assumes a position with the arches still present.

stated in an address to physiotherapists that habitual movement at a joint always has some conjunct rotation associated with it. He also pointed out that at every joint a bone moves in a curved line, and that every muscle is at some time or other a rotator.

## Degrees of freedom

Degrees of freedom is the term denoting the number of axes in which a joint may move. One degree of freedom occurs at the interphalangeal joints, and two degrees at the metacarpophalangeal joints where there is abduction and adduction in addition to flexion and extension. Three degrees of freedom takes place at the shoulder and hip joints only. The carpometacarpal joints of the thumb allow only two degrees of freedom as the rotation during opposition cannot be performed independently and is therefore conjunct rotation.

## Close-packing

Close-packing is a feature of synovial joints in which the joint surfaces fit together maximally in one position only. This occurs usually at one extreme of the available movement when the capsule and ligaments become taut and spiralised.

This close-packing produces joint compression, and no traction force is capable of separating the joint surfaces. It is a position which can take great strain by virtually making two bones act as one, but which has the disadvantage of being prone, in severe trauma, to injuries such as torn ligaments or even bone damage. It is dependent, therefore, on strong muscle power for the provision of additional stability and joint protection.

This is the most advantageous position in which to immobilise joints, especially those of the hand.

The ligaments, being maintained in a stretched position, are unable to contract adaptively, so that when any plaster or splint is removed the joint is easily mobilised. It is known as the 'safe' position of the hand. The wrist should be positioned in some extension, the metacarpophalangeal joints in about 70° flexion, and the interphalangeal joints in nearly full extension.

## Loose-packing

Loose-packing is the converse of close-packing, when the joint surfaces are no longer compressed and the ligaments and capsule are relaxed. It is in this position, where there is normally some 'play' in the joint, that the accessory movements should be performed, both for maintaining movement and for mobilising when the joint is stiff.

*Accessory* movements are the result of in-congruent joint surfaces moving one on another through the loose-packed range. They may occur during both active and passive movement as the result of an external distorting factor. It is the pass-ive accessory movements, however, of spin, slide, distraction and compression in which the physio-therapist has a particular interest for carrying out her mobilising techniques.

Joints should not be immobilised in their loose-packed position, unless there is joint disease. The slack ligaments and capsule will automatically contract, producing joint stiffness which needs many months of treatment to reverse. Metacar-pophalangeal joints which have stiffened in exten-sion are particularly difficult to mobilise sufficiently to recover full flexion.

## MOVEMENTS OF THE JOINTS

Movements are extremely complex and a basic description only is given in the following paragraphs.

## The wrist and intercarpal joints

The wrist is formed by the articulation of the radius with the scaphoid, lunate and triquetral, and the movements are intimately linked with those at the intercarpal joints.

Palmar and dorsiflexion, and radial and ulnar deviation take place at both wrist and intercarpal joints. There is in fact divided opinion as to whether it is mainly flexion or extension that occurs at the radio-carpal joints (Williams & Warwick 1980, Mennell 1971). A large proportion of the move-ment certainly occurs at the intercarpal joints.

Ulnar deviation takes place mainly at the radio-carpal joint but radial deviation, which has less range, is an intercarpal movement. Accessory movements include anterior, posterior and lateral gliding at both radio-carpal and intercarpal joints, with a considerable amount of axial rotation at the radio-carpal joint.

The wrist is close-packed when in full extension. It is usually easier to regain flexion than extension of the wrist following lengthy immobilisation in the neutral position.

## Carpometacarpal joint of the thumb

This is a saddle (sellar) joint formed between the trapezium and the first metacarpal. The shape of this joint is concave in one direction and convex in the other, and with the attachment of the ligaments, allows movement in flexion and extension, abduc-tion and adduction, circumduction and opposition. A small degree only of flexion can take place be-fore conjunct rotation occurs, which together with abduction produces opposition. This enables the pulp of the thumb to contact the finger tips. Axial rotation and distraction are the only accessory movements possible.

This joint is close-packed when in abduction and extension.

## Carpometacarpal (CMC) joints and the inter-metacarpal joints

These joints allow only very small gliding move-ments, which assist in the 'cupping' of the hand. The accessory function is in the spiral twisting of the metacarpals on the carpus.

## The metacarpophalangeal (MCP) joints

These joints are ellipsoid in shape allowing flexion and extension, abduction, adduction and circumduction. A small degree of conjunct rotation takes place, especially of the index finger with its ability to flex towards the palm and also to oppose towards the thumb (Fig. 1.16a & b).

Abduction of the fingers takes place maximally when the joints are extended, decreasing to minimal movement when the joints are flexed. This is due partly to the tightening of the collateral ligaments in the flexed position, and partly to the fact that the interossei have been pulled anteriorly and therefore can no longer effect abduction.

There are similar movements in the metacarpophalangeal joint of the thumb as in the fingers but of less range, especially abduction and adduction. Stability at this joint in the thumb is preferable to hypermobility, especially when normal carpometacarpal joint movement is present.

The MCP joints of the fingers are close-packed in flexion (Fig. 1.18) and the MCP joint of the thumb is close-packed in extension.

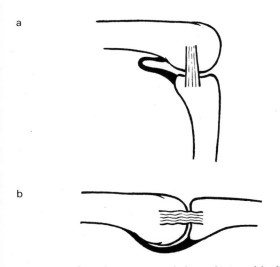

a

b

**Fig. 1.18(a & b)** The metacarpophalangeal joints of the fingers are close-packed in flexion and loose-packed in extension.

## The interphalangeal (IP) joints

These are hinge joints, allowing flexion and extension with some conjunct rotation. They are close-packed in extension.

*All metacarpophalangeal and interphalangeal joints* have accessory movements of anterior,

posterior and lateral gliding plus rotation and distraction.

## MUSCLE ACTIVITY

With the many articulations, and particularly the chain formation of the fingers, hand function requires a complex mechanism of muscle control. The combination of extrinsic and intrinsic muscle action enables the variety of movements to be achieved, with the usual interaction of prime mover, antagonist, synergist and fixator.

Broadly speaking, the long muscles produce gross finger movement whilst the small muscles provide power and stability. This is illustrated by a comparison of the slender hand of the artist or dancer with the squat and muscular hand of the labourer.

Flexion movements are the result of a simultaneous shortening contraction of the flexors together with a lengthening contraction of the extensors. Extension movements occur when the procedure is reversed. Both normally combine with intrinsic activity.

Greater knowledge has been gained from electromyographic studies which identify the co-ordinated muscle activity of the hand (Long 1968). A brief description follows of this muscle action.

### 1. Free flexion at the interphalangeal joints

This is mainly performed by flexor digitorum profundus (FDP). If no flexion is required at the distal interphalangeal joints, only flexor digitorum superficialis (FDS) contracts and it does this best with the wrist held in some flexion as seen in the hook grip (Fig. 1.7). Superficialis activity is most pronounced in the index finger, and is sometimes absent or underdeveloped in the little finger.

### 2. Flexion followed by extension at the metacarpophalangeal joints with the interphalangeal joints held fully flexed

This is brought about by the long flexors and long extensors, and not by any intrinsic activity. The intrinsics, however, must be capable of being fully stretched to allow this movement to occur.

### 3. Interphalangeal joint extension with simultaneous metacarpophalangeal joint flexion

This is performed by the interossei, and not the lumbricals as previously considered. It is an activity requiring large forces, partly because it is the converse of the relaxed position and partly because it stretches the capsular structure of the metacarpophalangeal and interphalangeal joints, as already discussed in the close-packed positions of those joints.

### 4. Full finger flexion followed by full finger extension

This is produced by the long flexors and extensors of the fingers. However, without simultaneous involvement of the lumbrical muscles there is a collapse of the multisegmental finger linkage (Landsmeer 1963). During movements of extension the strong visco-elastic property of flexor digitorum profundus prevents the full extension of the fingers by extensor digitorum communis unless there is intervention of the lumbricals. This can be seen in the combined median and ulnar nerve lesions at wrist level with resulting clawing, otherwise known as the *intrinsic minus* deformity. During extension movements it is the action of the lumbricals that slackens the tension of flexor digitorum profundus distally, thereby allowing the interphalangeal joints to extend.

*Clinical note.* In high median and ulnar nerve lesions, with FDP and FDS paralysed, EDC is able to extend all the fingers joints efficiently and without clawing.

### NEUROMUSCULAR CONTROL

Besides the normal neurophysiological control there are some specific factors relating to the hand.

1. *Motor units.* A great proportion of units are of a small innervation ratio, one cell innervating a few muscle fibres only, thus allowing precise movements to be learnt easily. This applies particularly in the small muscles of the hand.

There are mixed types of motor units in the flexor digitorum superficialis; the small units enable skilled movements, and the larger innervation ratio units ensure the muscle stamina needed for hook grip.

2. *The proprioceptive feedback* is highly efficient in the normal hand. The lumbricals are sometimes referred to as *sensory muscles* because they are particularly well supplied with annulospiral nerve endings, and they enable information to be relayed back to the cortex. The information includes the altering relationship of structures such as muscles and tendons to one another, and the speed of movements. This feedback assists in learning fast skilled movements, e.g. typing and playing musical instruments, and in all activities of the hand.

### SENSATION

Sensibility of the hand is a highly developed function in man and depends on the ability of the brain to interpret the impulses which it receives from both cutaneous and proprioceptive sources. The representation on the sensory homunculus is therefore proportionately higher for the hand than to a large extent the rest of the body.

Sensation must be adequate for us to perform our tasks efficiently. Any sensory deficit will reduce performance, and conversely any early difficulty in motor performance will reduce the development of full sensibility. Sensation, in fact, cannot be divorced from movement. It is therefore essential that both assessment and treatment of sensory problems are always considered together with function (Wynn Parry & Salter 1976).

### Sensory functions

The main sensory functions are:
1. Stereognosis, or the recognition of objects by palpation and manipulation.
2. Sensory feedback from all receptors. This is essential for ensuring a highly skilled and smooth performance of movement.
3. Protection, as the result of excitation of receptors by noxious stimuli
4. Orientation in space.

### Sensory modalities

Sensory stimuli are initiated as a result of excitation of the sensory nerve endings. Their source may be:

1. Exteroceptive, which includes the skin, ears, eyes and other internal organs.
2. Proprioceptive, from joint capsules, muscle spindles and golgi tendon organs.

## Cutaneous modalities

The skin of the hand has a particularly prolific supply of sensory nerve endings which act as receptors. The brain receives and interprets any differences between the impulses which have been generated by these specific receptors. Anomalies of the cutaneous distribution occur fairly frequently, especially of the radial nerve (Fig. 1.19).

The elementary cutaneous modalities are:

1. Light touch
2. Pain
3. Heat
4. Cold.

*Pressure* incorporates a combination of touch, stretch of skin, slight movement of joints and tendons, and stretch of muscle fibres. It therefore necessitates a complex form of judgment.

*Two point discrimination and localisation* are deductions which can only be made after some years of sensory experience. Both are incorporated together with the cutaneous modalities listed above.

Two point discrimination is the ability to recognise whether the skin is being touched by only one or by two points simultaneously. It is developed to a fine degree in the skin of the finger tips. It should be tested with a moving and not stationary two point touch as the receptors adapt to a stationary touch extremely quickly thus making it difficult to discern a stimulus.

Localisation is the ability to recognise the exact position of stimulus on the skin. It also should be tested with a moving touch.

As Wynn Parry pointed out in 1981 there has been a total change in the concept of physiology of sensation. It is now considered that there are not only specific receptors for each type of stimulus, but also that the receptors have varying thresholds of sensitivity to the different stimuli (Iggo 1984).

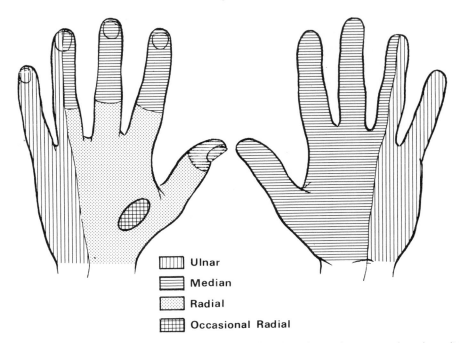

Ulnar
Median
Radial
Occasional Radial

**Fig. 1.19** Normal cutaneous distribution of median, ulnar and radial nerves. The median may replace the radial nerve distribution over the dorsum of the hand. Occasionally the radial nerve retains supply of a small area only at the base of the thumb web.

The discharges are then coded in patterns in the spinal cord and central nervous system. The cortex has the ability to interpret the variation of sensory stimuli received according to factors such as their frequency, intensity and duration in addition to their source.

## REFERENCES

Horton M E 1971 The development of movement in young children. Physiotherapy 57: 155–158

Iggo A 1984 Cutaneous receptors and their sensory functions. Journal of Hand Surgery 9-B(1)

Landsmeer J M F 1963 Co-ordination of finger–joint motions. Journal of Bone and Joint Surgery 45-A: 1654–1662

Long C 1968 Intrinsic–extrinsic muscle control of the fingers. Journal of Bone and Joint Surgery 50-A: 5

MacConnaill M A 1964 Joint movement. Physiotherapy 50: 11

Mennell J McM 1971 Manipulation of the joints at the wrist. Physiotherapy 57: 3

Williams P L, Warwick R 1980 Gray's anatomy, 36th edn. Churchill Livingstone, Edinburgh

Wynn Parry C B 1981 Rehabilitation of the hand. Butterworths, London

Wynn Parry C B, Salter M 1976 Sensory re-education after median nerve lesions. The Hand 8: 3

## FURTHER READING

Kapandji I J 1982 The physiology of joints, vol 1, Upper limb. Churchill Livingstone, Edinburgh

Napier J 1956 Prehensile movements of the human hand. Journal of Anatomy 89: 564

Tubiana R 1984 Examination of the hand and upper limb. Saunders, London

# 2

# Assessment

Loss of function in the hand following injury may result from a wide variety of factors. Immobilisation of the hand rapidly results in stiffening of the numerous small joints, and the adjacent structures easily become contracted and adherent and the tissues fibrotic. A thorough preliminary examination by the physiotherapist is essential, when any problems needing treatment can be identified and measurements recorded. By listening to the patient's comments, observing the hand and its movements and utilising the recorded measurements, an analysis of the cause of dysfunction can be made. This will enable the physiotherapist to decide on the priorities of treatment, and to devise an appropriate programme. Two patients with seemingly identical injuries may have different complications following surgery, and will therefore need totally differing treatment programmes.

Regular reappraisals should be made, either weekly or at suitable intervals, with further measurements recorded to monitor progress. Discussions among all members of the rehabilitation team, comprising surgeon, occupational therapist, physiotherapist nurse and social worker, are crucial for effective management. The patient needs to understand as much as possible concerning the mechanics of his hand, and the effects of the injury and the treatment planned: in this way he can be more involved in his own rehabilitation. His co-operation is essential if a satisfactory result is to be achieved.

This chapter gives a general outline of assessment. As so many variations are possible with a hand injury, each case should be assessed and

ASSESSMENT CHECK LIST

| Name | Date |
| --- | --- |
| Diagnosis | Dominance |
| Occupation | Leisure interests |
| *History* of injury and treatment<br>    Present problems, e.g. difficulty in certain activities, pain etc.<br>    Expectations and worries—social, psychological | |
| *Observation*: Scar or lacerations, position of hand and fingers, wasting, deformities,<br>    autonomic etc. Movement of hand | |
| *Palpation*: Scars, indurated areas, painful spots, flattening of arches, loss of elasticity | |
| *Measurement of movement*: Joints, webs, excursion, muscle chart | |
| *Sensation*: Cutaneous alteration, localisation, stereognosis | |

**Fig. 2.1**    Assessment check list.

recorded on an individual basis. Figure 2.1 provides a useful check-list of the assessment and the measurements which may need to be included. Further specific details may be found in the chapters dealing with particular conditions and injuries.

## REFERRAL

The referral from the surgeon or physician should include the following:
1. Diagnosis
2. Brief history of injury and surgery
3. X-rays
4. EMG reports (if any).

The full medical notes should be available for perusal.

## GENERAL OBSERVATION

A recently injured or post-operative patient who is needing physiotherapy may still be in bed with his hand in elevation. At a later stage he will be ambulant and attending the department. The first general observation can be made even when the patient's hand is still in elevation, or as he walks into the department. It should include:
1. General posture of hand (Fig. 2.2a & b)
2. Patient's attitude to hand, i.e. whether cheerful or depressed
3. His attempted use or protection of hand.

The physiotherapist should also observe the patient while he undertakes normal routine daily activities such as dressing or pulling out a chair. In

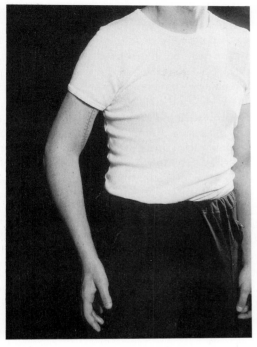 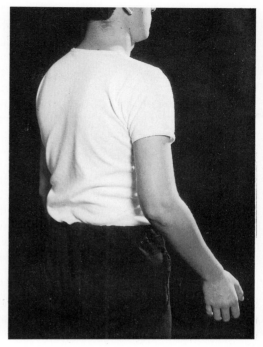

**Fig. 2.2(a & b)**   Abnormal posture of the hand. Note the increased supination and wrist extension and the decrease of finger and thumb flexion as the result of a high median and ulnar nerve lesion.

this way impressions may be formed both of the severity of injury and of the patient's attempt, if any, to cope with the disability. This visual assessment will give an indication of the patient's probable motivation and help the therapist to decide on the initial treatment.

## HISTORY

Information obtained from the patient is mainly subjective and this should include:
1. How, when and where the injury occurred and any background cause.
2. First aid, surgery and other treatment given.
3. Whether pain is still experienced and if so whether it is acute, from recent trauma and surgery, some residual discomfort, or constantly severe and intractable.
   The patient is asked for a description of his pain, but care should be taken that words are not put in his mouth.
   a. What type is the pain? Is it throbbing, shooting, burning, aching etc?
   b. Is it continuous or intermittent?

c. Does anything particular set it off?
d. Does anything relieve it?
The patient is asked to record his level of pain on the 10 cm line of a visual analogue scale, both before and after treatment (Fig. 2.3) (10 is the worst imaginable pain). A note is made of the

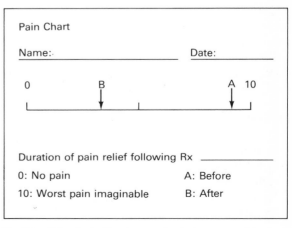

**Fig. 2.3**   Pain chart. The degree of pain is measured by the patient on a visual analogue 0–10 scale. 10 is the worst imaginable pain.

duration of any relief gained from treatment.
4. Employment, personal care and leisure activities. What he cannot do or is finding particularly difficult is recorded.

 If the injury is recent it may be impossible for the patient to identify the difficulties at this stage.
5. Any social problems should be identified and solved quickly as they detract from the patient's ability to concentrate and co-operate on treatment e.g.:
  a. Financial hardship with loss of earnings
  b. Family difficulties, e.g. care of young children whose mother needs treatment.
6. Expectations should be obtained. Does the patient understand the extent of injury, the time necessary for recovery and the probable outcome? Is he satisfied with treatment so far? What are his priorities and are they the same as the physiotherapist's?
7. Psychological factors. How much is the patient affected by and worrying about his injury and cosmetic effect? Will he need referral to a psychologist?
8. Compensation. This may have a bearing on his rate and degree of recovery by reducing his motivation.

## EXAMINATION

The position for examining the hand and the tempe- rature of the room should be comfortable for both patient and examiner.
1. Post-operatively or following severe injury the patient will be in bed with the whole arm in elevation.

 The patient's hand and arm should be supported on two or three pillows during the examination.
2. For ambulant patients, a pillow on top of a cantilever table is found to be most satisfactory. The table-top can be drawn up over the patient's knees even when he is in a wheelchair. The therapist is close enough to examine the hand easily, and the patient can see all that is happening, which is important.

## OBSERVATION

With both hands resting on the pillow, compare the affected side with the normal (Fig. 2.4a). Observe and record the following objective information.
1. *Oedema*
 Is the whole or only part of the hand affected (see also under measurements)?
2. Alterations in size.
 Is there loss of finger pulp and tissue bulk (Fig. 2.4b)?
3. *Scars*
 Are these from the original injury, incisions or skin grafting? Are they, because of their position and direction, likely to cause contractures? They can be recorded on an outline diagram of the hand.

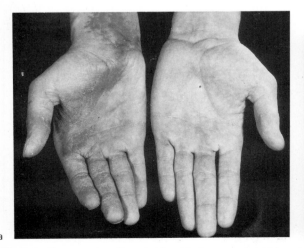
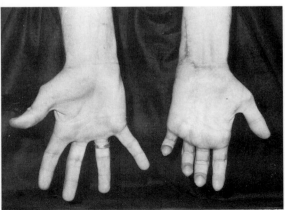

a    b

**Fig. 2.4** Compare the affected side with the normal. (a) Note the scar, the altered position of the thumb, the flexed and adducted position of index and middle finger and the sympathetic changes of the median distribution. (b) Note the loss of pulp on the affected side.

4. *Muscle wasting*
   Is this noticeable in:
   a. Forearm
   b. Thenar eminence
   c. Hypothenar eminence
   d. Interosseous spaces both dorsal and volar (Fig. 2.5)
   e. Thumb web space?
5. *Deformity*
   This may be due to skeletal damage, an imbalance of muscles, adherence of scars, circulatory damage or a nerve lesion. The following observations should therefore be made:
   a. Arches may be flattened
   b. Position of thumb may be flat beside index finger (Fig. 2.6), or contracted across palm.
   c. Position of fingers may be altered from normal, i.e.
      (i) A flexion deformity with MCP and IP joints held in more flexion than normal (Fig. 2.6).
      (ii) An extension deformity of MCP and IP joints with loss of usual flexor tone in fingers (Fig. 2.2).
      (iii) An intrinsic minus or claw hand deformity with MCP joints extended and IP joints flexed (Fig. 2.7).
      (iv) An intrinsic plus deformity with the MCP joints held in flexion and the IP joints extended. There are varying degrees of this deformity but when severe it is usually accompanied by some swan-necking of the fingers with prominent bases of the middle phalanges (Fig. 2.8).
      (v) A Swan-neck deformity, with the proximal interphalangeal joint held in hyperextension, and the distal interphalangeal joint held in some degree of flexion (Fig. 2.8).
      (vi) A boutonnière deformity with the proximal interphalangeal joint flexed and

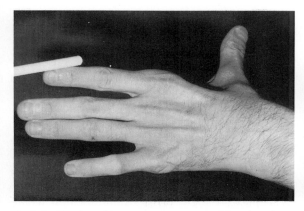

**Fig. 2.5** Wasting of interosseous spaces and thumb web.

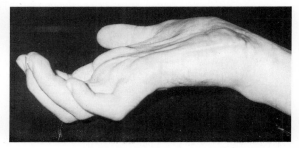

**Fig. 2.7** The claw deformity of a median and ulnar nerve lesion. Note the flattened arches and thenar eminince.

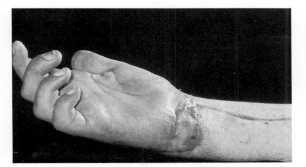

**Fig. 2.6** The thumb lies in a flattened position and middle, ring and little fingers are held flexed by adhesions at the wrist. The posture of the index finger is normal.

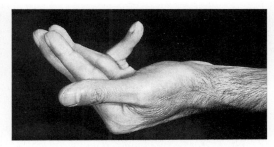

**Fig. 2.8** Severe intrinsic contracture illustrating inability to extend MCP joints. The little finger has been affected by a Volkmann's ischaemic contracture. Note swan necking of ring finger.

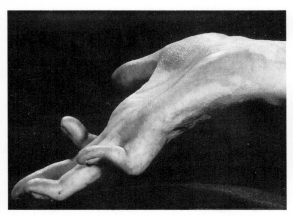

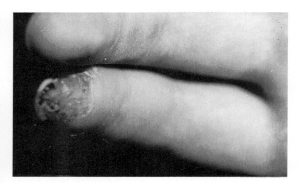

**Fig. 2.11** A trophic lesion.

**Fig. 2.9** Boutonnière deformity caused by severe extensor expansion damage from burns with a swan-neck deformity of the ring finger.

the distal joint hyperextended (Fig. 2.9). A mallet finger deformity with loss of active extension at the distal joint (see p. 121).
  d. Finger movements may produce drag on adherent scars.
6. *Condition of skin and nails*
  Can the following be observed, and if so do they follow a peripheral nerve or root pattern?
    a. Colour may be changed from normal, i.e. pinky-purple with loss of mottling (Fig. 2.10)
    b. Sweating may be absent or excessive
    c. Skin surface may be dry and scaly (Fig. 2.10)
    d. Skin texture may have become papery thin and shiny
    e. Trophic lesions or burns may be present (Fig. 2.11)

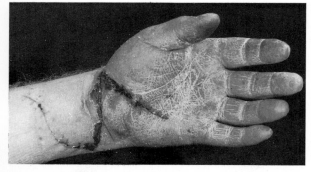

**Fig. 2.10** Skin colour may change and surface become dry and scaly.

  f. Hairs may be deformed due to follicle changes, or there may be excessive growth
  g. Nails may have become ridged and brittle.
  If these autonomic changes are present they will be similar in area to those described under the headings 'palpation' and 'sensory changes'

PALPATION

Sympathetic changes should be palpated using the fingers. The same area of skin should be found affected as that already observed.
1. Skin temperature may be cold or warm according to the surroundings.
2. Sweating may be absent initially or excessive later. The dorsum of the fingers should be used for palpation to avoid the normal tackiness of the therapist's own fingers.
3. Skin texture may develop a dry scaliness which later becomes shiny and papery thin.
4. Scars and adherence and the hard induration of tissues surrounding scars can be palpated with the finger tips.
5. Tissue elasticity may be altered. A 'woody' feel with loss of elasticity of the whole hand may be experienced when the therapist uses both her hands to manipulate the normally mobile structures. It is important for the patient to know that the rigidity of his hand is recognised.
6. A 'boggy' feel may be palpated with synovitis in the MCP joints and in the flexor tendon sheaths.
7. Painful areas may be identified. It is preferable to leave this palpation until the end of the examination.

## TESTING AND RECORDING OF MEASUREMENTS

Measurements need to be made in order to establish the effectiveness of the treatment and to monitor progress, to assess the value of the techniques used, and to provide information for the surgeon prior to any corrective surgery being performed.

### Standardisation of measurements

Standardisation of procedures is essential for results to be meaningful, but it is difficult to totally eliminate all variables. The following factors are prerequisites for the maximum standardisation of measurements.

1. The time of day should be the same. Early in the morning is often suitable as it eliminates any variation of activities immediately preceding measurement. (This is probably not suitable for rheumatoid arthritic patients.)
2. The position of the patient should be identical for repeat measurements.
3. The assessor should be the same wherever possible. There will always be slight variations between people's measurements, even when the techniques appear identical. If research is involved the assessor should not be the therapist treating the patient.
4. Daily activities and medications, if altered, can affect the measurements. Pain, for instance, can reduce both range and power of movement, as also may drugs and lack of sleep.
5. The decision whether to feedback the results or not must be made prior to measurement. For a purely objective assessment it is better not to tell the patient the results. Psychologically, however, the patient needs encouragement which the improving measurements can provide.
6. The equipment used should be calibrated where possible, to ensure consistency of readings.

### Recording

Standardisation of records is desirable nationwide, but it is essential in each department and is preferable throughout the hospital. Problem orientated medical records (POMR) can provide the uniformity needed. This method also eliminates the need for standardised

| Joints | | Date | | | Excursion movements | Date | | |
|---|---|---|---|---|---|---|---|---|
| Wrist | Fl/Ext | | | | Finger tips to wrist | | | |
| | Rad/Uln | | | | Finger tips to palm crease | | | |
| | Prop/Sup | | | | Finger tips away from wrist | | | |
| Ind | MCP | | | | Finger tips to table (extension deficit) | | | |
| | PIP | | | | Thumb web (Ind MCP to thumb IP jt) | | | |
| | DIP | | | | Web 2/3 | | | |
| Middle | MCP | | | | Web 3/4 | | | |
| | PIP | | | | Web 4/5 | | | |
| | DIP | | | | Total span | | | |
| Ring | MCP | | | | Thumb to index | | | |
| | PIP | | | | Thumb to middle | | | |
| | DIP | | | | Thumb to ring | | | |
| Little | MCP | | | | Thumb to little | | | |
| | PIP | | | | *Accessory movements found limited* | | | |
| | DIP | | | | | | | |
| Thumb | MCP | | | | Joints—1. | | | |
| | IP | | | | 2. | | | |
| | | | | | 3. | | | |

**Fig. 2.12** Measurements check list: joints, digit excursions and webs.

pro forma covering all measurements of the hand. One form, when totally comprehensive for all the complexities arising from hand injury, proves very unwieldy. Documents that relate to problems only are more compact and therefore more suitable. A check-list is given (Fig. 2.12) to ensure that no measurements are forgotten.

*The terminology* should be standardised and the following joint abbreviations used throughout:

| | |
|---|---|
| Carpometacarpal | CMC |
| Metacarpophalangeal | MCP |
| Interphalangeal | IP |
| Proximal interphalangeal | PIP |
| Distal interphalangeal | DIP |

*Rubber stamps* provide an outline of both aspects of the hand, and also the whole arm, which can be printed onto the documents (Fig. 2.13). They are found useful for recording the exact position of:
1. Scars
2. Localised painful areas
3. Sensory changes and incorrect localisation
4. Positioning of electrodes.

*Flow charts* should be used for the measurement of joint range, web spaces, overall finger movement, stereognosis, and for pain evaluation. Measurements recorded in columns are the easiest to follow when made over several weeks.

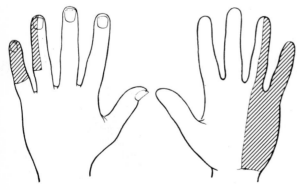

**Fig. 2.13** A rubber stamp of the outline of a hand provides an easy means for recording scars, areas of pain, and altered sensation. The shaded area shows anaesthesia following an ulnar nerve lesion at the wrist.

## Problem Orientated Medical Records (POMR)

These records which are part of the Problem Orientated Medical Systems introduced by Dr Weed in 1968, are a means by which improvement of medical communication, education and research may be achieved (Heath 1978). The standardisation of medical documents means that it is possible to carry out concurrent, even retrospective, patient care audits for quality assessment and technique evaluation (Bromley 1978).

POMR may be used by the whole multidisciplinary team, each discipline adding its own relevant material, or they can be used effectively by the physiotherapy department alone (Richardson 1979). They provide a system of documentation which is thorough, accurate and simplifies the handover of the patient's care from one staff member to another, as the problems needing attention are clearly identified.

POMR use four main headings for recording information as follows:
1. Data base
2. Problem list
3. Initial plan
4. Progress notes.

### Data base

This should include patient's name, age, occupation, hand dominance, employment and leisure interests. The diagnosis and clinical details should be recorded in this section.

### Problem list

This should include all the identified problems needing both physiotherapy and other treatment or assistance, which may be stiff joints and functional difficulties such as eating and dressing (Fig. 2.14). These should all be numbered and the problems should be indicated as active or resolved. The date on which they are resolved should be recorded.

### Initial plan

The initial treatment plan is drawn up by utilising the previously identified and numbered problems. A complete programme together with the detailed management of each problem is outlined using the same numbers. The patient should always be given an explanation at this stage and goals should be set regarding the degree and rate of recovery.

### Progress notes

These too are related to the already identified and

| Problem | Active | Date | Resolved | Date |
|---|---|---|---|---|
| 1 # | Shaft prox phalanx Lt index and middle fingers | 30.10.86 | K-wire | 31.10.86 |
| 2 | Oedema of index and middle fingers | 31.10.86 | Minimal | 10.11.86 |
| 3 | Stiffness MCP and IP jts | 3.11.86 | Minimal | 20.11.86 |
| 4 | Difficulty in dressing and buttons | 6.11.86 | No difficulty | 1.12.86 |

**Fig. 2.14** Problem-orientated medical records: the problem list.

numbered problems. They may be recorded diagrammatically as flow charts, with progress plotted daily or weekly, or they may be recorded in narrative (again either daily or weekly) in the form of SOAP notes as follows:

*S*ubjective information should include the patient's own account of the history and other relevant details such as pain.

*O*bjective information should include facts such as surgical procedures, and clinical observations such as measurements of joints and movements.

*A*nalysis of the present position, the cause of residual problems, and the short- and long-term goals should be made by the physiotherapist after having carried out a full assessment.

*P*lan of future treatment should be discussed concerning physiotherapy, occupational therapy, resettlement and return to work. An immediate programme of treatment should be arranged.

### Final discharge summary

The final discharge summary is an essential part of the progress notes. It relates back to the problem list, with a record of those problems which have been resolved and any which remain.

### VIDEO RECORDING

A video recorder in the department is a further means by which the patient's hand condition,

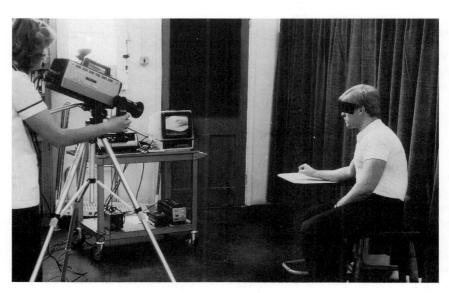

**Fig. 2.15** A video recorder provides a further method of recording hand activity.

movements and function can be usefully recorded (Fig. 2.15). It is surprising how quickly patient and therapist forget both the severity of the injury and its effect on function unless it is visually recorded. Trick movements in particular, which can be difficult to describe and record, are demonstrated effectively when using this equipment.

## TYPES OF ASSESSMENT

Assessments made by therapists are either functional or clinical. Both are necessary for good patient management.

### Functional measurements

Patients may find it impossible to perform functional tests initially, but they should be carried out as soon as they are feasible. These tests will be considered in more detail later in this chapter. Some of the difficulties that the patient is experiencing will already have been noted during history taking. The physiotherapist must consider the main functional problems carefully as they should influence the treatment programme. For example, emphasis can be put on increasing the range of a joint that has been identified as limiting the patient's functional performance. It is therefore essential that the findings of all assessments are utilised.

### Clinical measurements

Immediately post-operatively the urgent need will be to treat the patient, but measurements should be taken as soon as possible in order to monitor progress.

## OEDEMA

It is important to be able to show progress in the reduction of oedema, the degree of which is likely to vary during the day. It depends largely on the position in which the hand has been resting. The best time for measuring is early morning when there will be least effect from postural variations. Measurements should be taken over several days if they are to have real value, because it is difficult to be consistently accurate each day.

### 1. A tape measure or expanding loop measure

This is used round individual fingers at the level of the interphalangeal joints. Biro dots should be marked on the skin to ensure the same level of measurement daily. A tape can be used round the palm in similar fashion.

### 2. The ring measure

This was designed for use with rheumatoid joints and is the easiest and most reliable method for measuring the oedema of fingers at the level of the proximal interphalangeal joints. It uses a 0–10 scale (Fig. 2.16).

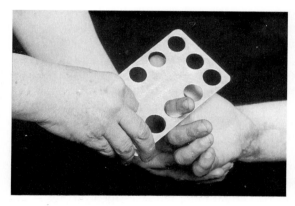

**Fig. 2.16** Oedema of the fingers measured at the level of the PIP joints using the 0–10 scale of the ring measure.

### 3. Water displacement

The whole hand is placed in a container already filled with water up to the overflow. A support inside the container ensures the identical position of the hand for each measurement. The amount of water which overflows into a container is measured accurately. This is not a suitable method to use if open areas are still present.

## RANGE OF MOVEMENT

All individual joint movements, the web spaces and the total excursion of fingers and thumb should be recorded. The latter may need to be combined with movements of the wrist. One whole hand movement of flexion and extension followed by opposition of the thumb towards the little finger will give an initial impression of the problems and of the detailed measurements which it is necessary to record.

### Individual joint measurements

Active, passive and accessory range should be measured. The shoulder and elbow joints should be checked for full movement, in comparison with those on the contralateral side. Movements of the wrist, i.e. flexion, extension, radial and ulnar deviation, and pronation and supination, should be recorded.

### 1. Active range

A goniometer is used over the dorsum of the fingers, and both flexion and extension are measured (Fig. 2.17a & b). Occasionally it is useful to record the resting position of the joint, e.g. when adherence is gross and is preventing normal movements, as occurs in tendon grafting of finger flexors. It is essential to be sure that the attempted movement is indeed different from the position of rest.

A small protractor, modified by rivetting a perspex pointer to the central pivot, makes a cheap and suitable goniometer. If the hand and fingers are swollen the goniometer should be placed on the line of the shafts of the bones, as measurements over the dorsum of the joints will vary with the oedema.

The individual joint range measurements are those described by the American Academy of Orthopaedic Surgery (1982), and both flexion and extension must be recorded. The degrees of movement can be added in brackets if desired, indicating any trend of alteration, but it is essential to know whether both the flexion and the extension are improving in order to give specific treatment.

### 2. Passive physiological range

If there is much discrepancy between the active and the passive physiological range the latter should also be measured and recorded. A different coloured ink used in the documents will help in comparing the two sets of measurements.

### 3. Accessory range

The motions of spin, glide and roll should be palpated as appropriate. The ten movements of the wrist of Kaltenborn (1980) is a useful guide (Fig. 2.18). An estimation of whether accessory movement is full, limited or nil should be recorded, or alternatively the 0–4 scale of Maitland (1977) should be used.

### 4. Odstock joint measurements

Both active and passive range may be recorded by this simple visual method of wire tracings. It is an alternative to the goniometer and is especially useful in the measurement of painful and severely deformed hands.

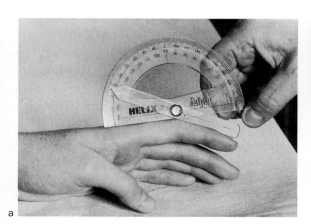
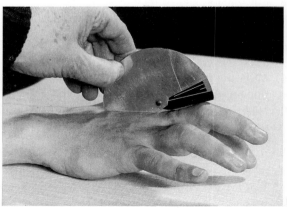

a
b

**Fig. 2.17** (a) This plastic protractor makes a cheap but accurate goniometer for measuring joints of the hand. (b) A small goniometer of this design allows hyperextension measurements to be made.

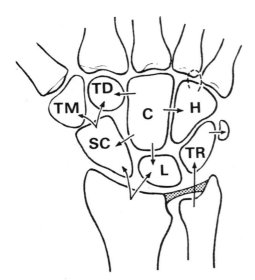

**Fig. 2.18** Kaltenborn's ten movements of the wrist.

A length of solder (170 mm long) is inserted into a clear flexible plastic tube. This combination of malleable solder and flexible tube facilitates accurate contouring of the finger without undue pressure. Spring wire is not suitable.

*Method*

a. Place the wire along the dorsum of the extended finger.
b. Gently adjust the shape of the wire until it exactly matches the contour of the finger (Fig. 2.19a). *Note* with a painful finger: bend the wire without making skin contact, then replace on the finger and check for accuracy. Repeat this until the correct contour is achieved.
c. Place the wire gently onto a piece of paper and trace the outline (Fig. 2.19b).
d. Mark the joints with an 'X'. Label them.
e. Repeat the measurement on flexion.
f. Superimpose the new shape on to an existing one, using the proximal phalanx as the BASE line (Fig. 2.19c).

Several tracings can be superimposed on each sheet by use of different colour pens or broken lines. All four fingers from one hand can be represented on one side of A4 paper. The thumb will require another sheet of paper.

## Total excursion measurements

Each individual joint may be fully mobile but total excursion of thumb and fingers from full flexion to full extension may be limited by weakness or by restriction of the soft tissues. A ruler from which the end has been removed as far as the nil reading, or a tape, can be used to measure the following:

1. *Distance of the finger tips towards and away from the palm*: An imaginary line from the medial end of the distal palm crease to the lateral end of the 'life line' crease is utilised (Fig. 2.20a & b). The wrist crease or a scar may provide a more suitable line for these measurements in the early stages when movement is severely restricted.

2. *Distance of finger tips from the table when the palm is uppermost*, i.e. extension deficit (Fig. 2.21). It is not possible to measure a gross flexion deformity by this method.

3. *Distance of thumb from the tips of fingers and from the base of little finger*, if opposition is reduced.

4. *Web spaces*. The thumb web should be measured between the MCP joint of the index finger and IP joint of the thumb (Fig. 2.22). This precludes measurement of any increasing lateral mobility of the index MCP joints. Individual finger webs can be measured between each finger tip.

Total span between tip of thumb and little finger should also be recorded (Fig. 2.23).

An alternative method of recording web spaces is to draw round them on to paper, and any alteration of space is added to the first drawing. This method, however, is not possible when flexion contractures are present.

5. *Salter measure*. After a radial nerve lesion the L-shaped measure with a scale on the short arm will show recovery of the wrist and finger extensors until they can contract through full range against gravity. The passive range of the joints should be full.

The forearm is supported on the table with the wrist held in the neutral position. The measure is placed in position over the arm, so that the finger tips are close to the scale (Fig. 2.24a). The patient is asked to lift his fingers up the scale as far as possible. Each finger tip is recorded separately as a negative reading.

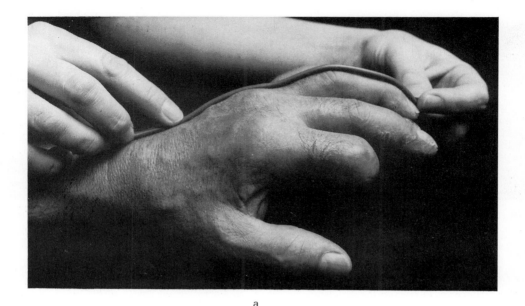

a

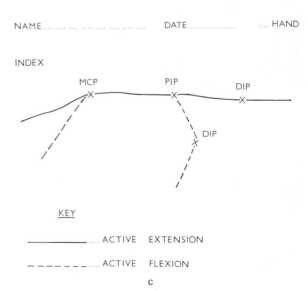

b

NAME.... .... .... .... .... ... ....        DATE.................        .... HAND

INDEX

MCP        PIP        DIP
X          X          X

DIP
X

KEY

_____ .... ACTIVE   EXTENSION

— — — — — .... ACTIVE   FLEXION

c

**Fig. 2.19**  (a) The shape of the wire is adjusted to the contour of the finger. (b) The outline is traced onto the paper and (c) superimposed onto an existing outline.

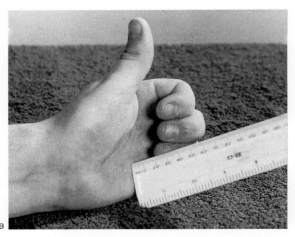
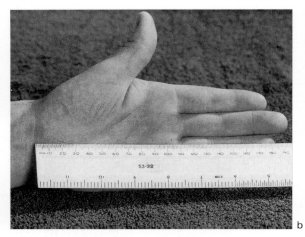

a
b

**Fig. 2.20** (a) Distance of the finger tips towards the palm. (b) Distance of the finger tips away from the scar, or the wrist crease.

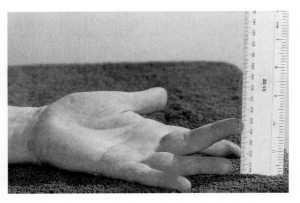

**Fig. 2.21** Distance of the finger tips from the table. This is the finger extension deficit, usually due to joint stiffness or adhesions.

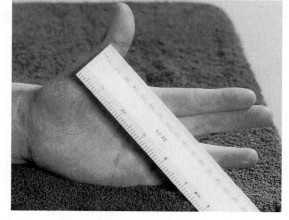

**Fig. 2.22** The thumb web should be measured between the MCP joint of the index finger and IP joint of the thumb.

When the patient is able to extend the fingers to the neutral position or possibly further, the measure is turned over and the forearm rested on top of it (Fig. 2.24b). The patient is again asked to extend his fingers and this time the wrist is allowed to extend also. Each finger is again recorded individually but with a positive reading.

6. *Presence of ischaemic contractures.* Direct injury to arteries or constriction from a tight plaster may cause ischaemic damage. This can lead to muscle contracture, and also the inability of the muscles to contract through full range.

a. Volkmann's ischaemia of the forearm prevents combined extension of wrist and fingers. As the

wrist extends the fingers will be pulled into a greater degree of flexion. Conversely the wrist has to flex to allow the fingers to extend. Occasionally the extensors may also be affected making it impossible to flex the fingers and thumb due to the contracture of the extensor muscles.

These contractures are difficult to measure. The proximal joints need to be stabilised in a standard position while a recording is made. The wrist should be held in a neutral position so that the measurement of the finger tips towards and away from the wrist crease can be read.

b. Intrinsic contractures of the small muscles of

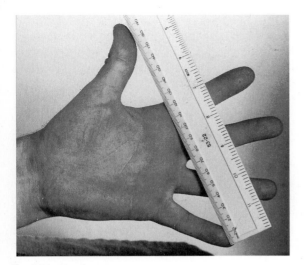

**Fig. 2.23**  Total span.

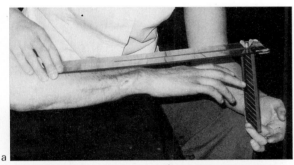

a

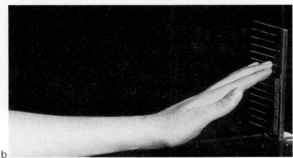

b

**Fig. 2.24 (a & b)**  Extensor deficit due to muscle weakness may be assessed using the Salter measure.

the hand are also difficult to measure. They may easily escape diagnosis altogether as they are not so obvious as a Volkmann's contracture. Nevertheless they can be extremely disabling, probably due to the additional proprioceptive loss. If the intrinsic 'plus' contracture is really severe it is poss-

ible that the patient will not be able to extend his MCP joints or flex his fingers.

The MCP joints should be extended into a neutral position, and the IP joints flexed, thus putting the small muscles on a stretch. A measurement of the distance of each finger tip towards the proximal finger crease should be made while the MCP joints are held in maximal extension.

If the thenar muscles are affected by an ischaemic contracture the thumb may be held in flexion across the palm. When this occurs it will severely interfere with the flexion of the index and middle fingers. The thumb web should be measured in both abduction and extension.

*Special note for measurements*

Care should be taken to ensure that any proximal soft tissue involvement is not producing a variable distal measurement. This is why a standardised position of the wrist joint is necessary when measuring total movement of fingers. For example, scarring and adherence of skin, tendons and subcutaneous tissue just above the wrist may limit the simultaneous extension of wrist, metacarpophalangeal and interphalangeal joints. If the wrist joint is flexed, however, the extension may be full in the other joints.

**Suggested sequence for measurement of joint range**

Not all previous measurements need to be recorded. When full active range is not possible the passive physiological movements of wrist and each joint of the thumb and fingers should be examined, taking care to relax any skin or tendon tension. The following sequence should help in the selection of appropriate measurements:

*When passive physiological movement is limited:*

a. Measure and record active movement.
b. Measure passive movement and record if it differs considerably from active range.
c. Examine accessory movement and record if limited by pain or stiffness.
d. Measure and record excursion of fingers and thumb from flexion to extension.

e. Measure the web spaces and record if less than unaffected side.

*When passive physiological movement is full:*

a. Measure and record the excursion of fingers and thumb from flexion to extension.
b. Measure web spaces and record if reduced from normal.

Measurement of individual active joint range is not appropriate when the passive movement is full, except following tendon surgery if adhesions in the flexor sheath are limiting finger movement. Progress can then be monitored by measuring the range at the distal interphalangeal joint.

## MUSCLE POWER

The normal interaction of agonist or prime mover with antagonist, synergist and fixator may be altered following injury, especially when nerve lesions are involved. To test muscle activity accurately the therapist should be familiar with:

1. Origins and insertions and any small slip attachments of muscles
2. General direction and diagonal in which each muscle lies
3. Relationship to the axes of the joints over which the tendon passes
4. Relationship with other muscles and tendons
5. Nerve supply and possible anomalies
6. The possible presence of trick movements.

### Types of muscle power assessment

The three types of tests for muscle power are:
1. The manual test of muscle groups
2. The manual test of individual muscles
3. The objective tests of grip and pinch grip strength.

The first two are tests which can only determine considerable differences in muscle power. It is essential therefore that objective tests using apparatus are performed as soon as possible.

The testing of group activity is especially relevant where muscles are expected to be weak from disuse, but otherwise normal. Individual muscle testing is essential to help diagnose and to monitor recovery following a nerve lesion and also for the selection of suitable muscles for transfer purposes (see p. 166).

Objective tests of grip and pinch are of greatest value when function is limited due to weakness of grip or pinch grip. The results of each test should never be considered in isolation but should be combined with the results gained from functional testing also.

## GROUP ACTION TESTS OF MUSCLES

All the proximal followed by the distal muscles should be tested. The patient is first asked to perform all shoulder and shoulder girdle movements (and neck if necessary), through full range, applying resistance at the same time. The distal joints should be tested following this. Movements should be graded as normal, slightly weak, or extremely weak etc.

## INDIVIDUAL MUSCLE TESTS

The muscles in the following description of tests are those acting distally to the elbow joints (see muscle chart, Fig. 2.25).

After a suspected or confirmed nerve lesion the following sequence of tests should be used:
1. Assess the muscles proximal to the lesion whose innervation is expected to be normal. Include shoulder and arm muscles. Weakness caused by disuse should be improved rapidly by exercise, and therefore can also be recorded by such terms as 'slightly weak' 'very weak' etc. If there is no muscle activity at all the cause will need investigation.
2. Assess the muscles distal to the lesion:
   a. Those likely to be unaffected by the lesion having an intact nerve supply. Check for normality or weakness.
   b. Those which have been affected by a nerve lesion. Check for both nil or any recovering activity, and for possible anomalies.

### Method of testing

Ensure that the patient is warm, comfortably positioned and supported, can see what is happening and understands the reasons for testing.

(i) Select the muscle and the joint movement required; test passively that the muscle has not

| Muscles of shoulder, upper arm and elbow, | | | Flexor carpi ulnaris | | |
|---|---|---|---|---|---|
| Supinator | | | Flexor digitorum profundus to ring and little | | |
| Brachioradialis | | | Abductor pollicis brevis | | |
| Extensor carpi radialis longus | | | Flexor pollicis brevis | | |
| Extensor carpi radialis brevis | | | Opponens pollicis | | |
| Extensor carpi ulnaris | | | Lumbricals 1 and 2 | | |
| Extensor digitorum | | | Abductor digiti minimi | | |
| Extensor indicis | | | Flexor digiti minimi | | |
| Extensor digiti minimi | | | Opponens digiti minimi | | |
| Extensor pollicis longus | | | Adductor pollicis | | |
| Extensor pollicis brevis | | | Lumbricals 3 and 4 | | |
| Abductor pollicis longus | | | Interossei dorsal | | |
| Flexor carpi radialis | | | Interossei volar | | |
| Palmaris longus | | | | | |
| Flexor digitorum profundus to index and middle | | | | | |
| Flexor digitorum superficialis | | | | | |
| Flexor pollicis longus | | | | | |
| Pronator teres | | | | | |
| Pronator quadratus | | | | | |

**Fig. 2.25** Muscle chart includes those muscles producing movement of wrist, fingers and thumb.

shortened adaptively and that the joint is mobile. Describe and demonstrate the action to the patient on both affected and unaffected sides. Give clear, simple commands.

(ii) Use any or all of the following:
  a. Isotonic prime mover action from outer to middle range which is usually the first to recover.
  b. Isometric contraction which sometimes is easier to teach to the patient, especially the intrinsic muscles (see p. 42). Again use outer to middle range at first.
  c. Synergic action. This occasionally may be identified before prime mover activity during early muscle re-innervation. For example, abductor digit minimi may first be felt to contract when opposing thumb and little finger towards one another.

(iii) Observe:
  a. The required movement, if any, at the selected joint.
  b. Any visible contraction of muscle and tendon.
  c. That no other joints are moving.

(iv) Palpate, when possible:
  a. The tendon close to insertion or along its length for any movement.
  b. The muscle bulk for any contraction.

(v) Facilitate by means such as muscle stretch, joint approximation or traction, the urging of the patient to produce or improve the movement, and application of resistance where suitable. The threshold of nerve conduction is raised following a nerve lesion and muscle activity will therefore benefit from this facilitation.

(vi) Record the muscle grade using the 0–5 Oxford scale (Medical Research Council 1981).
  0 No contraction.
  1 A flicker of movement. This is usually first palpated with the muscle contracting in its middle to outer range.
  2 A small range of active contraction, between middle and outer range, with gravity eliminated.
  3 Some movement against gravity, but the muscle is still unlikely to contract through full range.

4 A full range of movement against gravity with some resistance.

5 Normal movement and power as compared with the unaffected side.

A comprehensive anatomy book in the department is desirable.

*Caution*

Early resistance and stretch of damaged or sutured structures is contraindicated. A suitable time lapse should therefore be allowed before testing these stronger grades.

| Movement | Prime mover | Secondary action |
|---|---|---|
| *WRIST* | | |
| Wrist flexion | FCR, FCU, PL | FDP, FDS, FPL, APL, EPB |
| extension | ECRL, ECRB, ECU | EDC, EDM, EI, EPL |
| Ulnar deviation | ECU, FCU | |
| Radial deviation | FCR, ECRL (ECRB) | APL, EPB |
| *FINGERS* | | |
| MCP flexion | Interossei/lumbricals | FDS, FDP |
| extension | EDC, EI, EDM | |
| abduction | Interossei—dorsal | EDC |
| adduction | Interossei—palmar | FDP |
| PIP flexion | FDS | FDP |
| PIP extension | Intrinsic muscles and EDC | – |
| DIP flexion | FDP | – |
| DIP extension | Intrinsic muscles and EDC | – |
| *THUMB* | | |
| CMC | | |
| Palmar abduction | APB | Combination of OPP and APL |
| adduction | Add P | Combination of EPL and FPL |
| Radial abduction | APL, EPB | |
| opposition | OPP (with APB, FPB and Add P) | |
| MCP flexion | FPB | FPL |
| MCP extension | EPB | EPL |
| IP flexion | FPL | – |
| IP extension | EPL | APB, FPB |

**Fig. 2.26** Chart identifying joint movements and respective muscle action.

**Complicating factors and some suggested solutions**

1. Scarring and adherence may prevent full excursion of the tendon. Check the contraction proxi-

mal to the level of injury and palpate and observe scar when patient is attempting movement.

2. Muscles may contract unexpectedly.
   Check for nerve anomalies by using electrical stimulation. Stimulate directly the unaffected nerve at both wrist and elbow. Observe if that same muscle contracts.

3. Deformities may change angle of pull, therefore muscles may become inefficient.
   Check X-rays. Consider the effect that deformity may have on muscle function.

4. Sensory loss may make it difficult for the patient to feel what he is trying to do.
   Check that he can watch his own activity, that he is performing the correct movement with his contralateral limb and that he has several attempts to produce his best action.

5. Trick movements will usually be found with peripheral nerve lesions of the upper limb, as most patients will themselves have discovered the means to produce some type of movement. Therapists must be particularly observant to detect these movements.

6. Pain may be so severe that it totally inhibits muscle contraction. The pain must be treated first.

**Trick movements**

Doctors and therapists will have been taught the basic action of normal muscles and therefore can anticipate which movements will be lost as the result of a peripheral nerve lesion. Frequently, however, the patient can produce more joint movements than are expected (Fig. 2.27). These are called trick or compensatory movements and are classified in detail by Wynn Parry (1981). They can be divided, broadly, into three categories:

*1. Normal secondary muscle action and anomalous nerve supply*

Detailed anatomical knowledge is needed of origins and insertions of the multiarthrodal muscles, the direction in which they lie, and their relationship to the fulcrum of the joints over which they pass. For example:

a. The slip from abductor pollicis brevis (APB) which inserts into the dorsal expansion of the

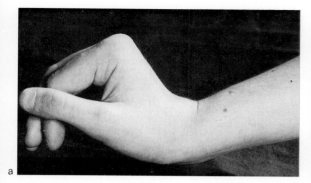

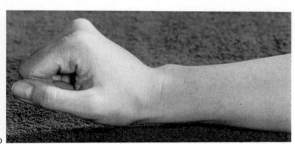

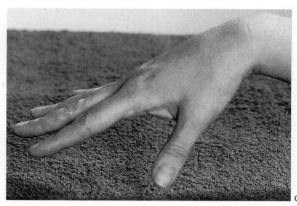

**Fig. 2.27** (a) This patient, with a high median and ulnar nerve lesion, is attempting to flex his fingers by tenodesis action. Note the extreme extension of his wrist as he attempts finger flexion compared with: (b) normal finger flexion with slight wrist extension and (c) normal finger extension with slight wrist flexion.

thumb, enables APB to extend the distal joint of the thumb when extensor pollicis longus is paralysed in a radial nerve lesion.

b. The forearm flexors and extensors can frequently provide a small amount of elbow flexion when the biceps is paralysed. This is because the origins of the common flexor and common extensor tendons are attached to the epicondyles of the humerus and thus proximal to the elbow joint. This is known as Steindler action and can be utilised in transfer procedures.

c. The position of abductor pollicis longus (APL), as it passes over the wrist joint, lies anterior to the fulcrum of the joint. Although it is grouped with the forearm extensors and abducts the thumb radially, it also flexes the wrist. In a combined high lesion of median and ulnar nerves, wrist flexion will therefore remain, produced by APL.

More details will be given with the individual nerve lesions of the expected trick movements which are due to these secondary muscle activities.

Anomalies of nerve supply can be misleading as they are present in about 15% of patients and they therefore make diagnosis more difficult. Nerve stimulation of an unaffected nerve may identify a possible anomaly, and this is important for correct diagnosis.

## 2. Pathological processes and surgical procedures

Denervation or ischaemia may frequently lead to a contracture of muscles. This can sometimes be used to advantage functionally when the antagonists are grade 4 or 5 Oxford scale. Although each joint may be mobile individually, the contracture will prevent full passive movement of all joints simultaneously, therefore the antagonist is also unable to move all joints through full range simultaneously. As the proximal joint is moved in one direction the distal joint will be moved passively in the opposite direction, and vice versa. This is known as tenodesis action. For example:

a. With high median and ulnar nerve or C7 brachial plexus lesions, the fingers will flex passively when the patient actively extends his wrist (Fig. 2.27a) especially if the flexors are contracted.

b. When active movement is present in wrist and finger flexors and absent in extensors as in a radial nerve lesion, finger flexion may produce passive wrist extension, especially if the extensors are contracted.

These movements can look realistically normal. In the past, by carrying out a surgical tenodesis, or tendon shortening procedure, function could be improved for the patient who was unlikely to gain further muscle re-innervation.

Careful note should be made of any tendon transfer procedures which have already been performed. Function can be improved by the re-positioning of muscles together with their neurovascular bundles (see p. 167). Muscles and tendons will then be lying in altered positions and directions and will therefore produce altered movements.

### 3. Deceptive movements

a. The effect of gravity can be utilised by the patient for demonstration purposes, but it is unlikely to provide a strong functional movement. For example, wrist flexion may appear to be present unless gravity is eliminated when testing. Similarly, elbow extension should only be tested with the effect of gravity eliminated.

b. Stabilising the distal joints and contracting the proximal muscles may give the appearance of activity at the middle joints. For example, with the therapist supporting the hand, the patient will be able to extend the elbow even though triceps is paralysed, by strong contraction of pectoralis major.

c. Rebound can result from relaxation of the antagonist muscles following their strong contraction and may look deceptively like a small contraction of the agonists, for example, attempted contraction of the fingers flexors after tendon surgery. If this is preceded by a quick extension movement, which the examiner can barely perceive, the relaxation can appear as a small flexion movement.

The paradox of trick movements is twofold. (1) The reverse action from that which is required frequently occurs. For example, in a radial nerve lesion, if the patient is asked to extend his MCP joints, the fingers will dip downwards. (2) There is movement at joints other than the one which has been selected. For example, in an ulnar nerve lesion, when asking the patient to abduct the MCP joint of his middle finger, the whole hand is moved from side to side on the fixed tips of the other three fingers. Abduction and adduction occur passively at the MCP joint of the other fingers, but there is no movement at the required joint.

Reduction of trick movement is frequently the first sign of early muscle recovery.

## ANTERIOR ANTEBRACHIAL MUSCLES

As a group these anterior forearm muscles may give slight assistance to elbow flexion, because the common flexor origin is attached to the medial epicondyle of the humerus, thus proximal to the elbow joint. They also have a mildly pronating effect when contracting together and most will assist in wrist flexion.

### Nerve supply

The ulnar nerve supplies flexor carpi ulnaris and the medial (ulnar) portion of flexor digitorum profundus. This is usually to both ring and little fingers, but occasionally to the middle finger also. The median nerve supplies the remaining muscles: pronator teres, flexor carpi radialis, palmaris longus, flexor digitorum profundus, flexor digitorum superficialis, and flexor pollicis longus.

### Testing position

Patient sits with forearm resting on a table, palm upwards.

### Flexor Carpi Ulnaris (FCU)

1. Rest hand, with wrist in some extension, over pillow.
2. Ask patient to flex wrist and to deviate in ulnar direction.
3. Palpate tendon immediately proximal to pisiform (Fig. 2.28).
4. Add resistance when suitable.

*Action.* Flexes wrist in combination with flexor carpi radialis. Ulnar deviates wrist with extensor carpi ulnaris. In isolation FCU produces diagonal movement of flexion combined with ulnar deviation. It contracts strongly as a synergist when opposing the thumb to the little finger.

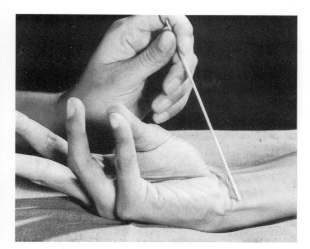

**Fig. 2.28** Flexor carpi ulnaris contracts strongly as a synergist when thumb is opposed to little finger.

## Pronator Teres (PT)

1. Rest hand in full supination over pillow.
2. Ask patient to turn his palm downwards.
3. Palpate muscle and observe for movement.
4. Add resistance when suitable.

*Action.* Pronates forearm from fully supinated to fully pronated position. Can become a strong elbow flexor especially in absence of biceps.

## Flexor Carpi Radialis (FCR)

1. Rest hand, with wrist in some extension, over pillow.
2. Ask patient to lift up his hand at wrist.
3. Palpate tendon immediately proximal to

scaphoid and lateral to tendon of palmaris longus (Fig. 2.29).
4. Add resistance when suitable.

*Action.* Flexes wrist in combination with FCU. Assists in radial deviation of wrist together with extensor carpi radialis longus and abductor pollicis longus. In isolation it produces an oblique movement of flexion combined with radial deviation.

## Palmaris Longus (PL)

1. Rest hand on pillow, wrist in neutral position.
2. Ask patient to flex wrist and while holding this position to oppose thumb to little finger.
3. The tendon of PL will be seen to stand out. (Fig. 2.30).
4. This procedure may be reversed, first opposing and then flexing wrist.

*Action.* Contracts palmar fascia and assists in flexing the wrist. PL is used as donor for both tendon grafts and transfers so that assessment of its presence is important.

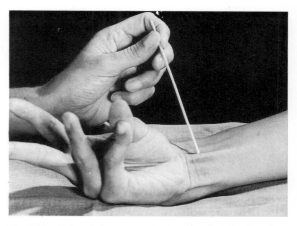

**Fig. 2.30** Palmaris longus contracts when first the thumb and little finger are opposed and second the wrist is flexed.

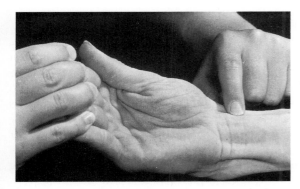

**Fig. 2.29** Flexor carpi radialis.

## Flexor Digitorum Profundus (FDP)

1. Rest hand on pillow with wrist in some extension.
2. Test each finger independently.
3. Support the middle phalanx.
4. Ask the patient to flex the finger tip (Fig. 2.31).
5. Observe movement at DIP joint.
6. Add resistance when suitable.

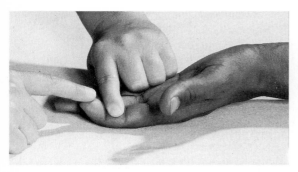

**Fig. 2.31** Flexor digitorum profundus tested with resistance.

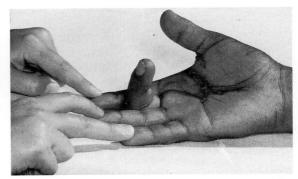

**Fig. 2.32** Flexor digitorum superficialis. Strength may be tested by resisting the muscle when the finger is already positioned.

*Action*. Flexes the DIP joints of the fingers. Assists in flexing PIP joints, MCP joints and the wrist.

### Flexor Digitorum Superficialis (FDS)

1. Rest hand on pillow, with wrist in neutral position and fingers extended.
2. Physiotherapist holds three finger tips in extension.
3. Ask patient to flex the free finger. If FDS is contracting the PIP joint will flex without any activity at the DIP joint (Fig. 2.32).
4. Gradually add resistance over the middle phalanx to test power and check that there is no action of FDP at distal joint.
5. Test each finger similarly. FDS to little finger may be absent.

*Action*. Flexes PIP joints of fingers, and following this it assists in flexion of MCP joints and the wrist.

### Flexor Pollicis Longus (FPL)

1. Rest hand on pillow with wrist in some extension, and thumb fully extended.
2. Support proximal phalanx.
3. Ask patient to flex the tip of his thumb.
4. Observe movement at IP joint and palpate tendon at insertion and over proximal phalanx (Fig. 2.33).
5. Add resistance when suitable.

*Action*. Flexes IP joint of thumb. Assists in flexion of MCP joint and wrist.

In absence of adductor pollicis action FPL combines with extensor pollicis longus to produce adduction

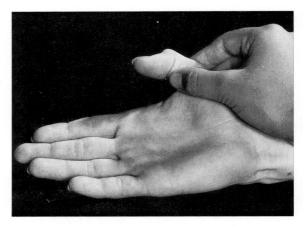

**Fig. 2.33** Flexor pollicis longus.

from the abducted position by reason of its diagonal direction over wrist and CMP joint.

## POSTERIOR ANTEBRACHIAL MUSCLES

These posterior forearm muscles, with common extensor tendon origin from the lateral epicondyle of the humerus, may have a similar effect to the flexors in assisting flexion of the elbow. This is quite frequently observed in patients with no activity present in the biceps, and is called the Steindler action. It may be utilised for tendon transfers to restore some flexion to the elbow by repositioning the origin more proximally.

## Nerve supply

The radial nerve supplies brachioradialis and extensor carpi radialis longus. The posterior interosseous branch then supplies supinator and all other extensor muscles of the group.

## Testing position

Patient sits with forearm resting on table, palm downwards (except for brachioradialis).

## Brachioradialis

1. Rest forearm in mid-position on pillow.
2. Ask patient to flex elbow.
3. Palpate muscle belly distal to the elbow joint (Fig. 2.34).
4. Add resistance if suitable.

*Action.* Flexes elbow in the mid-position. Assists both supination and pronation to the mid-position.

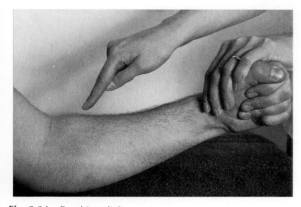

**Fig. 2.34** Brachioradialis.

## Extensor Carpi Radialis Longus (ECRL) and Brevis (ECRB)

1. Rest hand over a pillow with wrist in some flexion.
2. Ask patient to extend wrist.
3. Palpate ECRL on the thenar side of the base of 2nd metacarpal. ECRL is easier to palpate when the thumb is flexed across the palm (Fig. 2.35).
4. Palpate ECRB on the thenar side of the base of the 3rd metacarpal with the fingers in flexion.

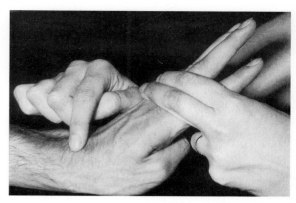

**Fig. 2.35** Extensor carpi radialis longus, palpated while the thumb is flexed across the palm.

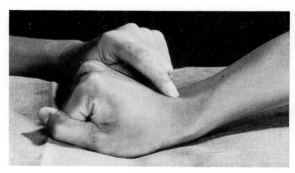

**Fig. 2.36** Extensor carpi radialis brevis can be palpated most easily when a strong fist is made.

*Action.* ECRL extends the wrist with radial deviation. ECRB provides straight extension of the wrist. It stabilises the wrist during gripping movements and can be palpated easily when a strong fist is made (Fig. 2.36).

## Extensor Carpi Ulnaris

1. Rest hand over a pillow with wrist in some flexion.
2. Ask patient first to extend wrist and ulnar deviate, and secondly to part fingers and thumb.
3. Palpate tendon immediately distal to ulnar styloid.

*Action.* ECU extends the wrist with ulnar deviation. It contracts strongly when all fingers and thumb are abducted (Fig. 2.37).

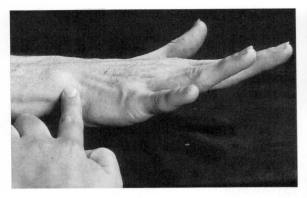

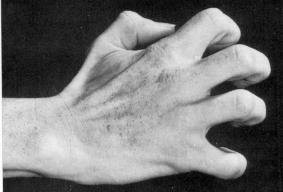

a

**Fig. 2.37** Extensor carpi ulnaris contracts strongly when all fingers and thumb abduct.

## Extensor Digitorum Communis (EDC)

1. Rest hand on pillow, wrist in neutral position and MCP joints in some flexion.
2. Ask patient to extend MCP joints, keeping IP joints flexed (Fig. 2.38a).
3. Ask patient to extend fingers at both MCP joints and IP joints (Fig. 2.38b).
4. Palpate tendon at level of wrist joint, observe both extension of MCP joints and contraction of tendons over metacarpals.

   *Action.* EDC extends MCP joints primarily, and IP joints only in conjunction with intrinsic muscles (Fig. 2.38b). It also assists in extension of wrist.

   *N.B.* Prevent wrist flexion when patient is attempting to extend his MCP joints.

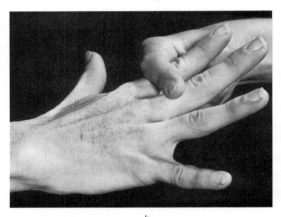

b

**Fig. 2.38** Extensor digitorum with interphalangeal joints: (a) flexed, (b) extended.

## Extensor Indicis (EI)

1. Rest hand on pillow with index MCP joint in slight flexion and middle and ring fingers in total flexion.
2. Ask patient to extend index finger and keep remaining fingers flexed.
3. Palpate tendon of EI (Fig. 2.39)
Positioning of remaining fingers in full flexion excludes activity of EDC.

   *Action.* EI extends MCP joints of index finger.

## Extensor Digiti Minimi (EDM)

1. Rest hand over pillow with little finger in slight flexion, and middle and ring fingers in total flexion.

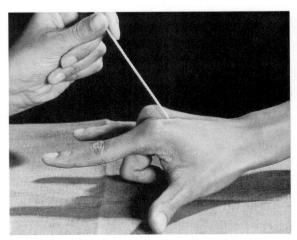

**Fig. 2.39** Extensor indicis should be tested with middle and ring fingers flexed.

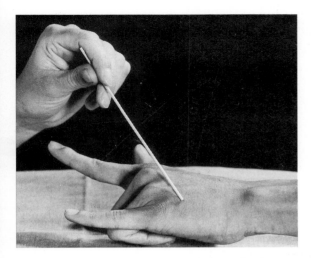

**Fig. 2.40** Extensor digiti minimi should be tested with middle and ring fingers flexed.

2. Ask patient to extend little finger and keep remaining fingers flexed.
3. Palpate tendon of EDM (Fig. 2.40).

Positioning of remaining fingers in full flexion eliminates activity of EDC.

*Action.* EDM extends MCP joints of little finger.

### Extensor Pollicis Longus (EPL)

1. Rest the ulnar border of the hand on pillow.
2. Ask patient to extend distal joint and lift whole thumb upwards, keeping it in the same plane as the index finger. Add resistance if suitable.

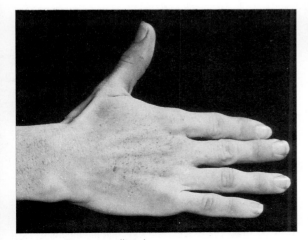

**Fig. 2.41** Extensor pollicis longus.

3. Palpate tendon and observe contraction of EPL on the ulnar side of the anatomical snuff-box (Fig. 2.41). Do not support the thumb for this test as it may cover up a trick movement.

*Action.* EPL extends IP joint of thumb, assists in extension of MCP, carpometacarpal and wrist joints, adducts and externally rotates the thumb column (into supination).

*N.B.* Interphalangeal joint extension of the thumb may be produced in a radial nerve lesion by abductor pollicis brevis (see p. 144). APB will at the same time, however, pull the whole thumb into palmar abduction with medial rotation.

### Abductor Pollicis Longus (APL)

1. Rest hand on pillow.
2. Ask patient to abduct his thumb.
3. Palpate tendon on radial border of anatomical snuff-box, volar to the extensor pollicis brevis tendon (Fig. 2.42).

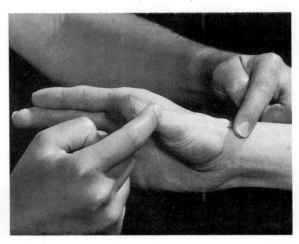

**Fig. 2.42** Abductor pollicis longus.

*Action.* APL abducts the thumb and radially deviates the wrist joint. It also assists in flexion of the wrist due to its slightly anterior position to the fulcrum of the joint. This action is evident with high lesions of median and ulnar nerves.

### Extensor Pollicis Brevis (EPB)

1. Rest hand on pillow

2. Place thumb in position with the IP joint flexed and MCP joint extended.
3. Ask patient to hold this position (Fig. 2.43).
4. Palpate tendon on radial border of anatomical snuff-box immediately dorsal to the APL tendon.

*Action.* EPB extends the MCP joint of the thumb. It is in action with all extension and abduction movements of the thumb, and assists in carpometacarpal extension.

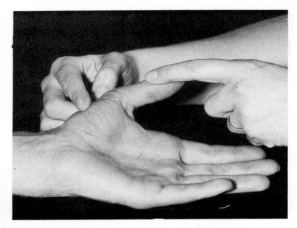

**Fig. 2.44** Abductor pollicis brevis abducts the thumb in a plane at 90° to the palm.

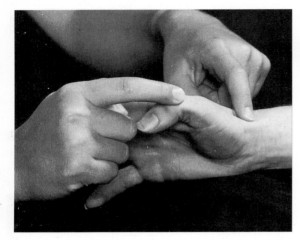

**Fig. 2.43** Extensor pollicis brevis.

## SMALL MUSCLES OF THE HAND

These muscles take origin distal to the wrist joint. The nerve supply is from median and ulnar nerves and there are frequent anomalies. The median nerve usually supplies abductor pollicis brevis, flexor pollicis brevis, opponens pollicis and the radial two lumbricals.

The ulnar nerve supplies the remaining two lumbricals, all interossei, abductor digiti minimi, flexor and opponens digiti minimi, the deep head of flexor pollicis brevis and adductor pollicis.

### Abductor Pollicis Brevis (APB)

1. Rest hand on pillow with palm upwards and thumb resting anterior to the index finger.
2. Ask patient to lift thumb upwards, at right angles to the plane of the palm. The thumb must not .drift into radial abduction.
3. Palpate muscle bulk close to the shaft of the 1st metacarpal (Fig. 2.44). Ability to hold thumb

away from close proximity to palm suggests some activity in muscle.

*Action.* APB abducts thumb at carpometacarpal joint into palmar abduction. It also assists extension of the IP joint of thumb because of its slip insertion into the dorsal expansion. It acts strongly to stabilise the thumb.

### Flexor Pollicis Brevis (FPB)

FPB arises from two heads. The deep is supplied by the ulnar nerve and the superficial by the median nerve.

1. Rest hand on pillow with palm upwards.
2. Position thumb with flexion of MCP joint and extension of IP joint (Fig. 2.45).
3. Ask patient to hold position and test MCP flexion with slight resistance.
4. Palpate immediately proximal to the MCP joint.

*Action.* FPB flexes the MCP joint, and assists in abduction and internal rotation of the thumb.

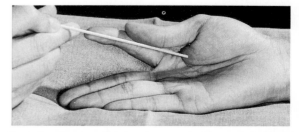

**Fig. 2.45** Flexor pollicis brevis. Note that the interphalangeal joint is extended.

## Opponens Pollicis (OP)

1. Rest hand on ulnar border with thumb in palmar abduction.
2. Ask patient to touch thumb tip to index finger tip and to rotate the thumb pulp to make contact with index finger pulp (Fig. 2.46).

*Action.* OP rotates the column of the thumb into pronation.

*N.B.* A combination of palmar abduction and MCP flexion, as in touching thumb tip to little finger tip, automatically produces conjunct rotation of the thumb. This can be misleading when assessing the opponens muscle.

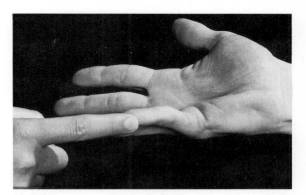

**Fig. 2.47**  Abductor digiti minimi.

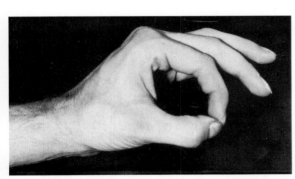

**Fig. 2.46**  Opponens pollicis rotates the thumb so that the pulp of both index and thumb contact one another. Opponens pollicis should not be tested with the little finger as conjunct rotation will automatically occur.

## Abductor Digiti Minimi (ADM)

1. Rest hand on pillow with palm upwards.
2. Ask patient to abduct his little finger with MCP joint in slight flexion (Fig. 2.47).
   Palpate muscle bulk.
3. Ask patient to oppose little finger to thumb
   Again palpate muscle.

*Action.* ADM abducts the little finger and helps flex the MCP joint from the fully extended to a slightly flexed position. It acts as a synergist during opposition of little finger towards thumb.

## Flexor Digiti Minimi (FDM)

This muscle assists in MCP joint flexion and in raising the fifth metacarpal head during opposition.

## Opponens Digiti Minimi (ODM)

1. Rest hand on pillow, palm upwards.
2. Ask patient to lift little finger towards the thumb (Fig. 2.48).
3. Palpate the muscle bulk volar to the ADM.

*Action.* ODM helps to raise and rotate the fifth metacarpal head for opposition of the little finger towards the thumb.

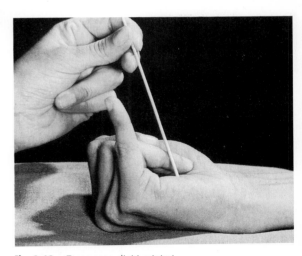

**Fig. 2.48**  Opponens digiti minimi.

## Adductor Pollicis (Add P)

1. Rest the ulnar border of the hand on pillow, with the thumb in palmar abduction.
2. Ask patient to adduct thumb to position anterior to index finger.

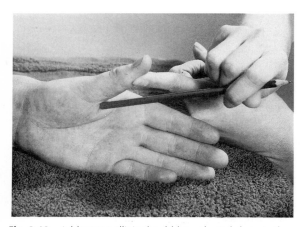

**Fig. 2.49** Adductor pollicis should be palpated deep in the thumb web from the volar aspect.

3. Palpate muscle deep in the web from the volar aspect (Fig. 2.49).
4. Observe for a smooth movement of adduction without pronounced thumb IP joint extension or flexion.

*Action.* Add P adducts the thumb at the carpo-metacarpal joint.

### Interossei: Dorsal (DI) and Palmar (PI)

The two actions of the interossei should be tested separately i.e. flexion of the MCP joints together with extension of the IP joints, and abduction and adduction of the fingers.

1. Rest hand palm upwards on the pillow with the MCP and IP joints in extension.

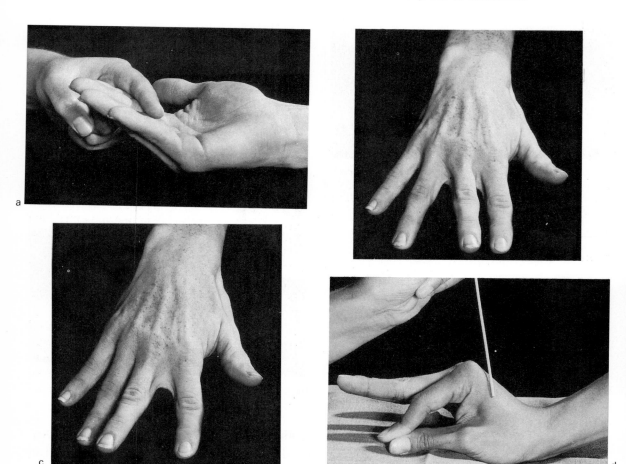

**Fig. 2.50** (a) Interossei maintaining flexion of the MCP joints together with extension of the IP joints. (b) & (c) Normal abduction of the middle finger in both directions. Note that the finger is held in slight extension while performing this movement. (d) 1st dorsal interosseous is essential for pinch grip.

2. Ask the patient to flex the MCP joints while keeping the IP joints in extension (Fig. 2.50a).

It may be easier for the patient if his fingers are placed in the required position and he is asked to keep them there, especially if at the same time the joints are given a quick approximation.

*Action.* Dorsal and palmar muscles contracting together flex the MCP joints and extend the IP joints simultaneously.

3. Rest hand with palm downwards on the pillow, with MCP joints in extension and some abduction.
4. Ask the patient to lift the middle finger, and while still lifted to move it from side to side (Fig. 2.50b and c).

After the middle finger the test is repeated on the ring finger. Resistance may be added if suitable.

Observe that movement takes place only at the MCP joint of the finger being tested.

Abduction and adduction of the index and little fingers can be misleading. When the interossei are totally paralysed some movement may be produced by alternate contraction of EI and EDC to the index finger. Similarly, abduction and adduction of the little finger may be produced by contraction of first EDM followed by EDC to the little finger.

The first DI should therefore be palpated when testing this movement of the index (Fig. 2.50d). Its activity is essential in providing stability for a pinch grip and for holding objects such as a pencil or a knife.

*Action.* With MCP joints in extension the dorsal and palmar interossei contract individually, producing abduction and adduction of the MCP joints. The interossei stabilise the fingers and the first DI is particularly important for pinch grip.

## LUMBRICALS

These muscles should be tested in conjunction with the long flexors and long extensors of the fingers as they normally act as a composite group.

1. Rest the flexor aspect of the wrist on a pillow, with the hand over the edge and the wrist in some flexion.
2. Ask the patient first to extend all joints of his fingers (Fig. 2.51) and then to flex them.
3. Observe during their movements that the fingers extend and flex normally, i.e. with no clawing

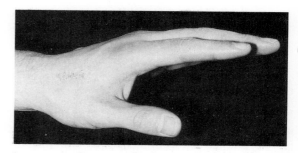

**Fig. 2.51** The lumbricals. Normal finger extension can only be achieved by a combined interaction of EDC and the lumbricals. Without lumbrical activity the fingers claw, making it impossible to hold the finger tips away from the palm during movement.

during extension and simultaneous movement of all joints during flexion.

*Action.* The lumbricals act as the controlling mechanism between long flexors and long extensors of the fingers. By releasing the strong pull of the flexors they prevent clawing. They are also very important as proprioceptors, relaying information such as speed of movements etc.

It is no longer considered that the position of MCP flexion with IP extension, which can be extremely strong, is produced only by the lumbricals, but that this is mainly the action of the interossei, assisted by the lumbricals. As the latter muscles both take origin from and insert into tendons it is also more logical that theirs is an adaptive and proprioceptive role rather than one of providing stability.

## OBJECTIVE POWER ASSESSMENT

Power is a good indicator of hand function and its measurement must form part of any hand assessment. There are several pieces of equipment available for this measurement. The modified aneroid sphygmomanometer is probably the most accessible, and the bag is comfortable for a patient to hold. It is also sufficiently sensitive to register weak readings. Conversely, dynamometers are often inflexible, and their hardness can produce discomfort with resultant muscle inhibition. They may also lack sensitivity for weak scores.

The most commonly measured aspects of power include gross grip, lateral grip or pinch and opposition pinch. There are many schools of thought on this topic and it is important to measure what is relevant and to standardise the procedures.

## Grip strength

The standard sphygmomanometer can only be used with patients who have less than 300 mmHg of grip strength, unless the column of mercury extends to beyond this figure. Research demonstrates that normal adult measurement ranges from 200 mmHg to 900 mmHg; therefore, to be useful, equipment must be capable of registering to this score. There are various other types of manometer available, where the pressure is expressed on a dial instead of a column. However, although the readings may go beyond the maximum of 300 mmHg, tests have shown that these are not as accurate.

The cuff (or bladder) of the aneroid sphygmomanometer, can be adapted by rolling and securing, so that when inflated, a constant circum-

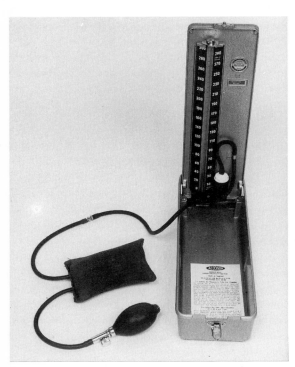

**Fig. 2.52** A standard aneroid mercury sphygmomanometer with a ready-made grip adaptation.

ference is achieved. The most common circumference sizes are 15, 18 and 20 cm (6, 7 and 8 in). However it is preferable and simpler to use a ready-made folded cuff sewn into a standard bag. These are often available from drug companies (Fig. 2.52). The ready-made bags can be inflated to variable amounts (10 mmHg, 20 mmHg, 30 mmHg etc.), but a common starting pressure is 20 mmHg.

### Method

Grip can be tested whilst the subject is sitting, standing or lying. The first position will be described here.

1. Sit the patient in a chair of comfortable height with the hips and knees at right angles and the feet on the floor.
2. The table height should be such, that whilst the patient is sitting with elbows resting on it, the shoulders should be neither elevated nor depressed. The forearm and hand should not rest on the table or lap.
3. The subject should grip the bag in the 'handshake' position, taking care not to press the bag against the body or the table.
4. On the command signal, but not before, the bag should be squeezed as quickly and as hard as possible and upon reaching the maximum, the subject should relax.

The result will indicate the rate of change of pressure, and speed of grip, but not the subject's endurance. Each test should be repeated (most commonly three times), alternating the hands to minimise fatigue. It is essential to take the maximum reading, not the average, as there is much variation amongst normals. Subjects may vary by as much as 100% during the day, thereby invalidating averages.

### Pinch grip

Pinch can be lateral, opposition or tripod. Since the surface contact between the measuring forces and the fingers is minimal, the equipment design is less critical than for testing gross grip. The method used to measure pinch may vary: some therapists adopt the previously mentioned bag used to test gross grip, while others use more specialised equipment such as a strain gauge. The same points itemised in the previous section regarding methodology still apply.

### Variables

Accurate readings are essential, but may be difficult to obtain when some types of apparatus are used. It is therefore advisable to use equipment which has a maximum hold facility, and which displays results on a digital display unit. The assessor may then concentrate entirely on the patient, making a special check for abnormal and compensatory movements.

The number of variables affecting the measurement of power are legion. They include: age, sex and posture; the position of the hand, its size and the direction of forces during gripping; the time of day and the environment; the psychological and general physical fitness of the patient and the fatigue and pain levels. Occupation and hobbies may influence strength, and the relationship of assessor and patient may affect the results.

Additional variables are caused by the material of the bag and the manner in which it is folded, its 'ballooning' when squeezed and the leak of air at pressures above 500 mmHg. This method should not be considered sufficiently reliable to compare one test with one undertaken the following week, and should therefore be used in conjunction with tests using strain gauges wherever possible. With returning power the patient should be asked to squeeze the different-sized bulb grips of the dynamometer, and use the pinch, opposition and lateral grips of the intrinsicmeter when this is available.

Studies have shown wide variation amongst normal subjects. Therefore it is irrelevant to compare a patient to a calculated average score. Similarly, judgements should not be made from a single reading. It is essential to look at trends, not absolute values. In the evaluation of the impaired hand the strength of the unaffected hand should serve as the most accurate reference. In bilateral conditions, however, no such control will exist.

Some studies of hand dominance have shown the dominant hand to be generally the strongest, whilst others indicate no significant difference. The latter appears to be the most commonly found conclusion, and this supports the use of the un- affected hand as a control whenever possible.

## SENSATION

Knowledge that sensation is normal, absent or altered will help both to confirm the diagnosis and to recognise that any reduced sensibility will be affecting the patient's hand function. Following the initial assessment any changes that occur may also indicate that nerve regeneration is progressing and that sensory re-education should be commenced. Monthly sensory testing and charting should then be undertaken.

Touch, localisation, stereognosis, proprioception and Tinel are of value for the therapist to test. Moving two point discrimination is an academic means by which sensory recovery may also be assessed. Pain should already have been assessed (p. 17).

It is useful to know how the patient views his sensory changes with regard to his function, and for him to show quickly on his own hand the area of any alteration, but the therapist must make her own observations separately.

The patient should be blindfolded during testing as many patients will be tempted to have a peep unless prevented. A mask or a folded triangular sling will make a suitable and comfortable blind- fold. The author prefers not to use a screen with a hole for the arms as psychologically it cuts off the patient from his task.

### Touch

This tactile test is used to identify whether the skin is anaesthetic, hyperaesthetic, hypoaesthetic or normal which will give an indication of the degree and stage of nerve involvement and recovery.

For the therapist this is performed most normally and practically by using the light touch of a finger tip. Extremely careful support should be given under the patient's hand so that the touch cannot produce any joint movement. He is asked to say immediately he feels the touch. In the area that he recognises light touch he should be asked whether or not it feels normal, and to describe how it is differ- ent, e.g. pins and needles, or cotton wool sensation. Occasionally an area of such hypersensitivity that it is painful even to light touch may be found follow- ing nerve injury, particularly brachial plexus involvement. This is known as hyperpathia.

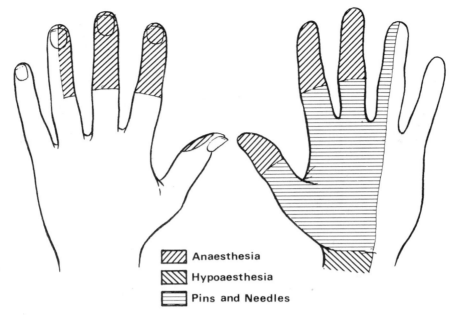

**Fig. 2.53** Progression of sensory recovery following a median nerve lesion. Different colours denote the variations and a legend is used for their identification.

The variations of both dorsal and volar surfaces are drawn on to the stamped diagram of a hand, and anaesthesia, hyperaesthesia, hypoaesthesia and acute hypersensitivity are shown in different colours. A legend is used for easy identification of these colours (Fig. 2.53).

Temperature and pin prick can also be tested if considered relevant to the patient's occupational and leisure activities. The areas are likely to be similar to those of light touch.

### Localisation

This test is used for discovering whether the patient can correctly identify the exact position of touch. It will indicate any need for re-education.

Localisation may be altered following nerve suture, due to crossed re-innervation, when the sensory neurones have been unable to regenerate to their correct end organs. Testing can only be carried out after some sensation has returned.

Two identical outline charts of the hand are used. The first is numbered in sequence over the affected sensory area and any incorrect localisation is charted onto the second using the sequenced numbers (Fig. 2.54a). With the patient's eyes closed a small area of skin is touched briefly, making a slight movement of the finger on the skin, which prevents adaptation of the nerve endings. The patient is then asked to open his eyes and point to the exact spot which was touched (Fig. 2.54b). This is done to prevent him feeling around for the spot. The position that he indicates, if incorrect, is referenced from the first chart and that number is recorded onto the second chart at the point of the therapist's touch (Wynn Parry 1981).

As the patient's efficiency improves, and he can localise correctly but slowly, the number of seconds' delay should be recorded on the chart. This is repeated at monthly intervals until his recognition is instantaneous.

### Stereognosis

This test is to discover whether and how quickly patients can identify objects and materials.

Testing should be performed only when some sensation, preferably normal, has returned to the finger tips. If hyperaesthesia is strong it is more difficult for the patient to differentiate between objects.

Large wooden blocks of varying shapes and

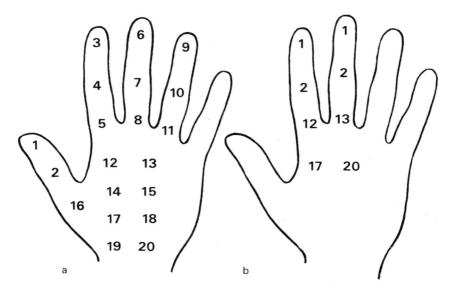

**Fig. 2.54(a & b)** Localisation. Areas are numbered in sequence on the left hand chart. (a) The position that the patient indicates, if incorrect, is referenced from the left chart and recorded on to the right hand chart, at the point of the therapist's touch (b).

weights give the blindfolded patient a preliminary introduction to stereognosis testing. The therapist should ask leading questions concerning the shape, size, angles and material that he is feeling. The time is recorded in seconds for correct identification and then the patient is asked to judge the weight of the blocks and put them in order.

Thirty selected everyday articles are divided into three groups of ten, of large, medium and small sizes (Fig. 2.55). Those for men should be different from those for women. Each is handed to the patient for identification, commencing with the largest. The time for correct recognition is recorded in seconds (Fig. 2.56). Anything incorrect is marked by a cross (X) and 'don't knows' by a dash (—). The patient is not told whether he is right or wrong, and is not shown the articles at the end of the test so that his memory will be involved as little as possible at the next testing session.

If he succeeds in identifying most of the large articles, he is tested with the medium, and then with the small. He should not be given the smaller ones if he had difficulties with the preceding group. Once a group has been commenced, however, it should always be completed.

It has been found necessary to include this large number of objects in order to reduce the memorising effect. For the same reason, testing should only be repeated at 4–6 weekly intervals or longer.

**Proprioception**

Total proprioceptive loss is extremely disabling. It is experienced usually with a combination of high median and radial nerve lesions, when the patients complain frequently of dropping the articles that they are holding. An ulnar nerve lesion, with intrinsic muscle involvement, may also reduce proprioception severely.

Joint position sense is tested by the physiotherapist giving a very slight movement of either flexion or extension and asking the patient to state in which direction the movement is occurring. The finger should be held on either side so that there is no increase of pressure in the moving direction and the patient must have his eyes closed or be blindfolded.

It can be tested more functionally by using a variation of thicknesses of a material such as wood. Small blocks should be graded for a minute increase in thickness (Fig. 2.57).

**Tinel test**

The level of sensory nerve regeneration and the site of the injury can be estimated by using the

| Large objects | | | Medium objects | | | Small objects | | |
|---|---|---|---|---|---|---|---|---|
| | Date | | | Date | | | Date | |
| Beer mat | | | Biro | | | Button | | |
| Bottle | | | Bulldog clip | | | Cork | | |
| Electric plug | | | Can opener | | | Drawing pin | | |
| Handle bar grip | | | Match box | | | Key | | |
| Nail brush | | | Nut and bolt | | | Marble | | |
| Scissors | | | Pencil | | | Paper clip | | |
| Screw top | | | Playing card | | | Rubber | | |
| Shuttlecock | | | Sparking plug | | | Rubber band | | |
| Tennis ball | | | Spanner | | | Safety pin | | |
| Tin box | | | Tape measure | | | Screw hook | | |
| *Textures* | | | *Coins* | | | *Timed tests* | | |
| E.g. Carpet | | | E.g. 50p | | | E.g. Blocks in board | | |
| Tweed | | | 20p | | | Weight of blocks | | |
| Velvet | | | 2p | | | Thickness of wood pieces | | |

Recorded in seconds        Don't know—        Wrong X

**Fig. 2.55**  Stereognosis testing. A variety of articles for testing should include objects in everyday use, materials and coins.

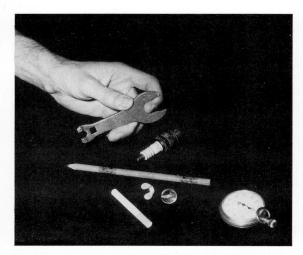

**Fig. 2.56**  Correct recognition of articles should be timed in seconds.

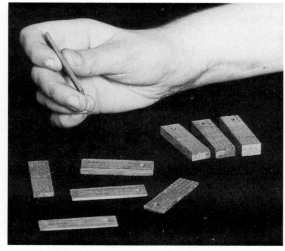

**Fig. 2.57**  Joint position sense may be tested functionally by putting different thicknesses of wooden blocks in order.

Tinel test (Henderson 1948), but this test should only be considered a probable and not an infallible indicator.

The therapist taps along the course of the nerve from distal to proximal. Pins and needles felt in the sensory distribution of the nerve will be experienced by the patient when the tapping reaches the site of nerve regeneration. If the tapping is continued proximally the sensory discharge may increase when the site of maximum regeneration is reached. The exact position at which this occurs should be measured in millimetres from a suitable bony point or skin crease. If the tapping is then performed from proximal to the estimated position of lesion, and continued in a distal direction towards the lesion, the exact site will be discovered by the intense degree of paraesthesia experienced by the patient.

The test must be carried out in the order suggested due to the carry-over of the sensations experienced. The distance between the two points and the comparison of strength of the discharges will indicate the degree of regeneration, and the rate at which it is occurring.

### Other forms of sensory testing

Cutaneous sensation may be tested by stroking a different diameter of monofilament, such as suturing material, lightly over the skin and asking the patient to indicate when he feels it. This is a very time consuming test but one which may, for the surgeon, indicate the extent of nerve regeneration. It does not, however, relate to the degree of functional sensation which the patient may regain. For this reason stereognosis and localisation are considered more practical forms of testing.

Two-point discrimination (Fig. 2.58) is similarly a test which does not indicate the patient's functional ability. If tested it should be performed using a moving touch (Dellon 1984).

Return of sensory conduction can be detected within a few weeks of commencement of nerve regeneration by using a simplified form of EMG apparatus. This technique is now being used for monitoring sensory nerve recovery following surgery. A sweatmeter also may be used to detect any return of sweating, which is an indication that recovery is occurring in the sympathetic nervous system.

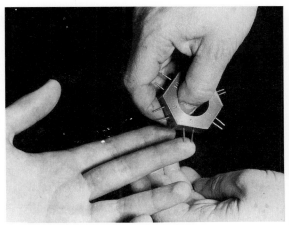

**Fig. 2.58** Two-pt discrimination, if tested, should be performed using a moving touch.

### FUNCTIONAL ASSESSMENT

Hand assessment must have a functional component and should be related to the everyday needs of the individual, according to his lifestyle. Power, anatomy and sensation do not alone reflect the true ability of the hand, as deformity and dysfunction are not always inseparable. To the patient with gross deformities, a fused joint, however abnormal, may be a stabilising influence. Functional deformity may thus be an important part of the analysis for hand effectiveness.

The hand, unprompted, assesses for temperature, weight and texture, and no assessment, game, activity or piece of equipment will relate this to individual and meaningful requirements. Where relevant, assessment should therefore include a functional analysis although this can only be subjective. One such system involves a chart which is jointly completed by both patient and assessor.

### Functional chart

This chart comprises a list of everyday tasks from which the patient selects the ones most pertinent to him. Against these he rates the degree of difficulty with which he performs the tasks. This is done by the patient marking the appropriate column, graded as either easy, fair, difficult or impossible. In bilateral conditions, where hand function may not be comparable, the letters R and L are used to denote

| Function | Easy | Fair | Difficult | Impossible | Reasons | | | | | | | | | |
|---|---|---|---|---|---|---|---|---|---|---|---|---|---|---|
| | | | | | 1 | 2 | 3 | 4 | 5 | 6 | 7 | 8 | 9 | 10 |
| | | | | | | | | | | | | | | |

**Fig. 2.59**  Functional assessment chart headings.

right and left hands. Where there is varied functional level due to active disease, it may be necessary for more than one form to be completed. The total number of functions selected may be inconsistent as not all individuals drive, have hobbies, or perform the same number of domestic activities.

Upon completion of these four columns, they are totalled up by the assessor to give a functional score. The therapist, together with the patient, then analyses reasons for difficulty by the selection of appropriate factors from a problem index.

## PROBLEM INDEX AND ANATOMICAL ANALYSIS

The 10 point problem index (Fig. 2.60) acts as a checklist for the assessor, and its numbers correspond to the 'Reasons' section. Having selected one or more causes for difficulty from the index, these numbers are ticked in the reasons columns. The problem index, however, can only be meaningful if it is qualified with the appropriate information (such as which hand or specific joint is affected).

Once the reasons columns are completed, they are also totalled. It is then possible to give both a functional score and to establish the reasons for difficulty, which if put in order of importance to the patient, provide the anatomical analysis.

1  Weakness

2  Pain

3  Thumb problems

4  Interphalangeal joint problems (IPJ)

5  Metacarpophalangeal joint problems (MPJ)

6  Sensory problems

7  Tendon problems

8  Wrist problems

9  Other joint problems

10  Other reasons

**Fig. 2.60**  Basic problem index.

## Examples of functional charts, scoring and problem indexes

Figure 2.61 shows a sample chart for a child or student, and Figure 2.62 shows an example of scoring. How this latter would be presented is now shown below:

PATIENT A

Total number of functions tested = 42.

**Functional score**

Easy = 2/42      Fair = 6/42      Difficult = 25/42
Impossible = 9/42

Hand dominance: R = Right Hand
                  L = Left Hand

Patient's name ...................................................................

Address .............................................................................

...........................................................................................

*How difficult are the following?*

Date .......................................................

| | EASY | FAIR | DIFF | IMPOSS | REASONS | | | | | | | | | |
|---|---|---|---|---|---|---|---|---|---|---|---|---|---|---|
| | | | | | 1 | 2 | 3 | 4 | 5 | 6 | 7 | 8 | 9 | 10 |
| *DRESSING* Buttons (large/small) | | | | | | | | | | | | | | |
| Zips | | | | | | | | | | | | | | |
| Shoelaces | | | | | | | | | | | | | | |
| Fastening clothes at back | | | | | | | | | | | | | | |
| Socks/stockings/tights | | | | | | | | | | | | | | |
| Tie | | | | | | | | | | | | | | |
| *TOILET/WASHING* WC | | | | | | | | | | | | | | |
| Taps | | | | | | | | | | | | | | |
| Wringing out flannel | | | | | | | | | | | | | | |
| Towelling dry | | | | | | | | | | | | | | |
| Holding soap | | | | | | | | | | | | | | |
| Cleaning teeth/using t'paste | | | | | | | | | | | | | | |
| Combing hair | | | | | | | | | | | | | | |
| Washing hair, back of neck, back, legs | | | | | | | | | | | | | | |
| Getting in/out of bath | | | | | | | | | | | | | | |
| *EATING/CUTLERY* Using a knife and fork | | | | | | | | | | | | | | |
| Holding a cup/saucer or mug | | | | | | | | | | | | | | |
| Lifting cup to mouth | | | | | | | | | | | | | | |
| Cutting meat | | | | | | | | | | | | | | |
| Holding a plate | | | | | | | | | | | | | | |
| *DOMESTIC* Making tea/coffee (pouring) | | | | | | | | | | | | | | |
| Unscrewing lids | | | | | | | | | | | | | | |
| Using tin opener | | | | | | | | | | | | | | |
| Making sandwich | | | | | | | | | | | | | | |
| Making toast | | | | | | | | | | | | | | |
| Cutting loaf | | | | | | | | | | | | | | |
| Washing/wiping up | | | | | | | | | | | | | | |
| Cooker controls | | | | | | | | | | | | | | |
| Ironing | | | | | | | | | | | | | | |
| Making bed | | | | | | | | | | | | | | |
| Washing clothes | | | | | | | | | | | | | | |
| *SCHOOL/COLLEGE* Writing | | | | | | | | | | | | | | |
| Typing/Computer | | | | | | | | | | | | | | |
| Using a ruler | | | | | | | | | | | | | | |
| Using a calculator | | | | | | | | | | | | | | |
| Geometry equipment | | | | | | | | | | | | | | |
| Slide rule | | | | | | | | | | | | | | |
| Drawing/painting | | | | | | | | | | | | | | |
| Books (holding, turning pages, carrying) | | | | | | | | | | | | | | |
| *HOBBIES* (e.g. Games: Toys: Skills) | | | | | | | | | | | | | | |
| | | | | | | | | | | | | | | |
| *GENERAL* Scissors | | | | | | | | | | | | | | |
| Using a door key | | | | | | | | | | | | | | |
| Door handles | | | | | | | | | | | | | | |
| Handling money | | | | | | | | | | | | | | |
| TV/radio/stereo | | | | | | | | | | | | | | |
| Telephone | | | | | | | | | | | | | | |
| *OTHER FUNCTIONS* (e.g. Transport) | | | | | | | | | | | | | | |
| TOTALS: | | | | | | | | | | | | | | |

**Fig. 2.61** Hand function chart for child/student.

| Function | Easy | Fair | Difficult | Impossible | REASONS | | | | | | | | | |
|---|---|---|---|---|---|---|---|---|---|---|---|---|---|---|
| | | | | | 1 | 2 | 3 | 4 | 5 | 6 | 7 | 8 | 9 | 10 |
| TOTALS | 2 | 6 | 25 | 9 | 20 | 18 | 10 | 7 | | | | | | |

**Fig. 2.62** Examples of scoring.

**Hand tested RIGHT (DOMINANT)**

*Reasons for difficulty/anatomical analysis*

1. WEAKNESS — Grip strength only 40 mmHg (20/42).
2. PAIN — Pain and hypersensitivity over scar site (18/42).
3. THUMB — Cannot perform opposition pulp/pulp pinch, lateral pinch grip only (10/42).
4. IPJ — Index finger, 15° flexion only, limiting pulp to pulp pinch grip (7/42).

**Sample problem index for an acute hand injury**

1. Weakness—Not yet attempting power functions.
2. Pain—When hand not elevated (see visual pain analogue).
3. Thumb problems—Traumatic amputation at level of metacarpophalangeal joint; no functional opposition.
4. IPJ problems—Cannot oppose/grasp as only 15° flexion at present.
5. MCP problems—Movement impeded by oedema (see item 10).
6. Sensory problems—Hand anaesthetic, glove distribution.
7. Tendon repairs.
8. Wrist problems—Wrist in flexed position (15–50°), no active extension yet.
9. Other joint problems.
10. Other reasons—Hand oedema impeding movement (measured by water displacement in perspex tank at 2.00 pm daily); unaffected (control) hand—350 cc; affected hand —420 cc.

**Case study**—Pre- and post-operative functional assessment in pollicisation of the dominant thumb

The patient whilst at work sustained a traumatic amputation of his dominant thumb and index finger, at the level of the metacarpophalangeal joints. Hand assessment was thus requested to ascertain the degree of difficulty imposed by the loss of the thumb, in both work and social life. The surgeons presented several options: to leave the hand alone; to cleft down to the carpometacarpophalangeal joint of the thumb and so provide a short but mobile stump for opposition and grip purposes; to perform radical surgery and either graft onto the thumb or pollicise using a finger or toe; to provide the patient with a prosthetic thumb.

An occupational therapist performed a detailed assessment which included a workshop analysis and job simulation during which the patient was tried both with and without a basic thumb post (Figs 2.63a and b). Following this, a report was taken with the patient to the combined hand clinic, where further discussion took place with the hand surgeons. In this instance it was concluded that the patient could not successfully change his hand dominance and that a normal length thumb was essential for the safe execution of his job. It was also recommended that for several reasons a prosthesis would not be satisfactory in this case.

The patient, having been assessed as being sufficiently motivated for the intensive rehabilitation programme that would follow, went for surgery and had a pollicisation of his great toe (Fig. 2.63c). A follow-up assessment revealed that not only was he able to return to work following this, but that his balance was not adversely affected, and he resumed soccer training with youth teams.

## WORK ASSESSMENT AND RESETTLEMENT

Employment is as important psychologically as it is financially, and with some exceptions, patients are

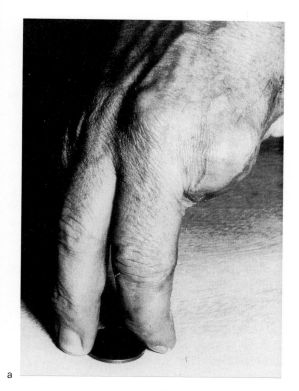

a

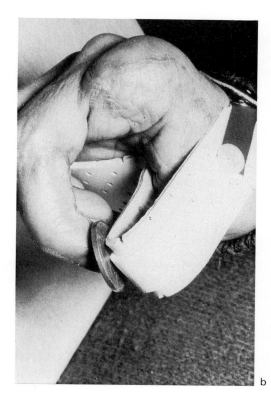

b

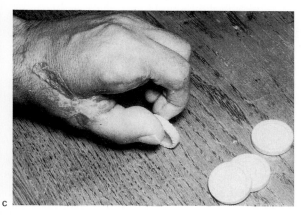

c

**Fig. 2.63** (a & b) The patient attempts a job simulation both with and without a basic thumb post; (c) Following pollicisation.

open and whether meanwhile he is financially secure. It is not unusual to find firms that have no sick scheme for employees.

## STAGE ONE: THE JOB DESCRIPTION

At the onset of treatment planning, a discussion should take place, in which a comprehensive job description should be obtained from the patient. This will not only assist in the planning of treatment, but also will serve to reinforce to the patient that his eventual re-employment is the ultimate aim of his rehabilitation programme.

From the job description, it will be possible to ascertain the skills that will be essential for the earliest possible return to work. A full assessment of work potential must then be done. Where severity of injury will prevent return to former employment,

anxious not only to keep their jobs, but also to return to them as soon as possible. Unfortunately in this age of job insecurity and high unemployment, prolonged time off work can mean redundancy. For the already unemployed, there is the added worry that a serious hand condition may exclude them from the open employment market. All these factors must be considered by the therapist as anxiety will adversely affect progress. It is therefore wise to check whether the patient's job is still consideration for retraining will be essential to maintain morale and to motivate rehabilitation. At the end of the day, it will be a combination of therapy input and patient effort that produces the desired result. The patient's awareness of his role is therefore vital.

## Guidelines for the job description

This should be divided into a general and a specific check list. The general section should include the following sub-headings:

### Occupation

The job title and a basic description of the post should include the name of the employee and relevant qualifications held.

### Conditions for employment

Is the job still open? For how long will it remain so? Will the employer offer an alternative (such as lighter duties) on a temporary or permanent basis? Would any change in duties involve a move to a different part of the company and possibly to another site? How would this affect the employee?

### Hours of work

This should include details of various systems such as flexi-hours, rotas, bonus schemes, and whether overtime is voluntary or compulsory.

### Length of service

Note how long the patient has been employed and ascertain whether this will influence his conditions for employment. Employers may be more flexible if an employee has been in the company for a reasonable amount of time. Also check whether the current post is bound by a time limit.

### Benefits

Check about the availability of sick pay and the rates. Also enquire about paid leave and when full pay actually commences.

### Health and safety

Enquire about the firm's attitudes to health and safety and its accident rates and sickness levels. Compare these with the patient's own attitudes.

The specific check list should be divided into physical, mental and general sections.

*Physical section should include the following:*

1. Whether the job is light or heavy and how much lifting is involved.
2. The specific movements and muscles required and the need for accuracy in those movements.
3. How much dexterity and hand–eye co-ordination is necessary and whether speed is an essential requisite.
4. The need for accurate sensation.
5. Whether the job requires bilateral arm and leg movements.
6. The senses involved.
7. The usual working position adopted, any changes or modifications that may be made and the length of time that the person must spend in that position (Fig. 2.64).

*Mental* section should, where appropriate, cover the following areas: numeracy skills, comprehension, communication, concentration and memory. In addition, note whether the post involves decision-making, problem-solving and the use of initiative. It is also important to ascertain the perceptual skills required plus the level of intelligence and training necessary for the job. Awareness of these aspects is essential should the hand condition dictate a change of employment whether temporary or permanent.

*General* section should include information such as whether the job is in or out of doors and whether it is classed as clean or dirty. If the latter applies, note if oil, water or grease is involved. Check the temperature of the environment, the machinery, tools, materials used (including chemicals), plus special handling procedures, use of protective clothing, safeguards on equipment, and health and safety measures. It may also be advisable to enquire about material or waste disposal if this is part of the employee's job. Other aspects to include in the conditions of work are the variety of work offered, whether there is good supervision and guidance, satisfactory industrial relations, good interpersonal relationships and management structures. Check if the firm offers break or rest periods and also if the job involves unsocial hours and on-call service. These latter points are particularly important where fatigue may be a consideration in safety and accident prevention, and if the patient has to drive. They may also dictate a longer period away from work

following hand trauma. Finally, it is worth checking on job satisfaction, boredom, motivation, reward and chances of promotion. Inability to work at speed may adversely affect reward or promotion chances and boredom and poor motivation may be detrimental to concentration and therefore safety, in addition to inhibiting effective and speedy rehabilitation.

## STAGE TWO: PLANNING

Following clarification of the patient's job requirements, assessment and treatment for return to the previous level of function are the major aims.

The following attributes should be considered with regard to fitness for work:
1. Skill
2. Strength
3. Endurance
4. Joint flexibility
5. Speed of action.

With a serious hand injury, the initial assessment should also consider the following points:
1. Will any disabilities hinder the patient?
2. Will he still be able to do his job?
3. What work suits him?
4. What are his aspirations and potential?
5. Can he be retrained?
6. Is he willing to be retrained?

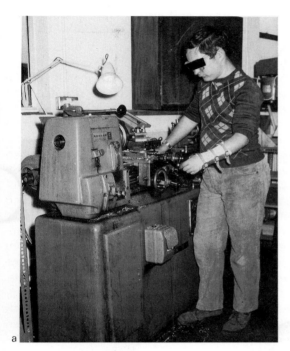

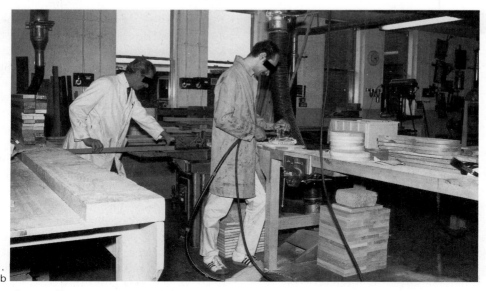

**Fig. 2.64(a & b)**  Work assessment in a rehabilitation workshop.

*Points to note*

Always be aware that hand injury can cause great emotional trauma and loss of mental equilibrium. Conversely, initiative and personal relationships can affect the disability.

If the injury was an industrial one, the patient may understandably be sensitive to thoughts of a return to the same working environment. It may therefore be necessary to liaise with both the patient and his employer in the early stages. In some cases, a visit to the actual place of work will enable the therapist to get a clearer idea of what the patient's job actually involves.

When the seriousness of the injury dictates that the patient will not be able to return to his previous job, the employer may offer alternatives, which may or may not be acceptable to the patient. However, if the employee can continue by using adaptations to his tools or equipment, the employer may be happy to support this.

## Compensation claims

Therapists have been known to state that patients with a compensation claim pending, are slower to respond to treatment. However, the claim of 'compensationitis' as the cause of slow recovery, despite intensive therapeutic intervention, is a grave accusation. Therapists, no matter how well intentioned, will find their attitude and response to the patient quite biased by this 'diagnosis'. There are many reasons for slow response to treatment, and of the non-physical ones, anxiety and depression are more likely than reluctance. The patient should always be given the benefit of the doubt and there should be no labelling unless the case is proven.

## Disablement Resettlement Officer

The Disablement Resettlement Officer (DRO) is the link between the hospital, patient and employer. Based in the local Job Centre, this person is responsible for the negotiation of employment for the registered disabled. Patients can make their own appointment to see the DRO at the Job Centre, although a DP1 form is necessary, bearing a doctor's signature, if retraining is to be required. This form gives the training centre the relevant medical and functional information that they require, before commencing assessment of suitability for retraining.

## PSYCHOLOGICAL ASPECTS OF THE IMPAIRED HAND

The psychological effects of hand impairment are considerable, irrespective of aetiology or severity. The hand is not merely an organ of function, it is an incredibly complex and highly evolved structure, capable of great acts of power one minute, yet the next, registering the finest of sensations whilst performing the most dextrous of movements.

Hand gesture is a vital adjunct to both verbal and non-verbal communication, and as such forms part of normal conversational practice. When silence is required, deafness or excessive noise prove a barrier to the voice, gestures become essential and complete conversations are conducted entirely by hand signs. Hand gestures may be friendly or unfriendly and can reflect mood or body tenseness, the so-called body language. Aside from essential communication skills, dance and mime would be infinitely poorer without hand movements.

To further evaluate the importance of the hand, there is need only to look at the frequency with which the word appears in language, and how often it is linked with beauty (for example handsome).

Without hand function, the traditional greeting of the handshake is lost. Character may even be judged by the style and firmness of the grasp offered. In society, there are secret hand signs and salutes, both indicating membership of a specialised peer group, to which the accurate execution of that sign is all important. This is found in both childhood and adult life.

Consciously or not, people observe others' hands, the gestures, position, condition of the skin, the nails and jewellery. The condition of the hands, and type and amount of jewellery worn, can reveal much of the individual's status, class and lifestyle. There is a ring for almost every occasion, and a meaning behind even the finger to be adorned. Reaction to the condition of a hand often tempers reaction to its owner. Well-manicured, clean hands are expected in certain professions (of either sex), and yet in other groups, this would be socially unacceptable.

People are at the mercy of their hand skills, as clumsiness is rebuked, yet skill is praised. However, the vital skill is still that of touch, either as a reprimand or as an expression of comfort, empathy, love or acceptance. There is frequent reference to the need for eye contact and yet simple touch can 'speak volumes'. Anxious or frightened patients or relatives are markedly reassured by touch, babies are soothed by it, and stroking helps relieve tension. Conversely, firm gestures or actual strikes are equally effective, the power behind the movement varying, dependent upon whether the intention is to threaten or to inflict actual pain.

The hand is the 'eye' of the blind and yet it is so often used similarly by the sighted. Using sight alone, palpation and percussion are invalid, the carpenter cannot accurately judge his finishes, the adult will not select one object from many in a trouser pocket nor the child find a marble in a sand pit.

The owner of a maimed or deformed hand is therefore deprived of many things. It is only fitting, in consequence, that the person be allowed a period of mourning in which to grieve this loss. The proportion of this reaction may bear little or no relationship to the cause or even extent of the injury. Complete loss of the hand may cause enormous problems in communities where amputation is punishment for crime. This latter point is also important in reconstructive procedures.

The hand is a device with many varied functions, and manipulative skill and power alone do not even begin to reflect the complexities of its skills. It vitally influences powers of investigation, expression and communication. Impairment can therefore cause great emotional trauma and disturbance of mental equilibrium, from which some persons may never recover.

## ANALYSIS OF PROBLEMS AND PLANNING OF TREATMENT

An analysis of the assessment findings is made firstly to identify the reason for the hand dysfunction, secondly to decide the means by which this dysfunction may be corrected, and thirdly to monitor progress during treatment.

The information which should be available for this analysis includes:
1. Diagnosis and brief surgical history, with dates.
2. X-rays which identify bony injury and joint involvement.
3. Early report from the ward of patient's general condition.
4. EMG report which may identify nerve degeneration or early re-innervation of muscles. It may show slowing of sensory and motor conduction rates. It can identify the occasional functional paralysis by showing that, although there is no voluntary movement, when the nerve is stimulated a normal muscle response is elicited.
5. Physiotherapy assessment.
6. Functional assessment from OT department.
7. Social workers and psychologist's report (if any).

## CAUSES OF LOSS OF FUNCTION

Some of the causes of disability to consider include oedema, pain, joint stiffness, skin adherence and loss of movement.

### Oedema

It may splint hand and fingers so rigidly that:
1. The tension makes it impossible to flex.
2. Any attempt at movement is very painful.
3. Fibrosis occurs causing loss of suppleness in the soft tissues, and flattening of the arches. A stiff non-functional hand results.

### Pain

This may be sufficiently severe that it will inhibit normal movement.
1. Pain following either surgery or injury is expected. It normally resolves itself within a few days.
2. Prolonged pain may be due to lengthy immobilisation or over-protection.
3. Severe intractable pain may follow peripheral nerve damage or plexus lesions. It may also result from a minor injury which develops into algodystrophy (otherwise known as reflex sympathetic dystrophy, or Sudeck's atrophy, see p. 136).

## Adherence of skin and tethering of tendons and muscles

This prevents full excursion of muscles, thereby reducing movement. It can lead to contractures and the joints becoming stiff if not correctly treated (see following paragraph).

## Stiff joints

These may be the result of:
1. Lengthy immobilisation in POP's etc., especially if immobilisation was in unsuitable position (see p. 10).
2. Intra-articular fractures, fractures close to the joint, or dislocations.
3. Contractures of skin, and adherence of scars, skin and tendons, preventing full range of movement.
4. Adherence of tendons in their sheaths.
5. Paralysis of muscles with loss of full movement, due to a nerve lesion, possibly resulting in contractures and stiff joints if the passive mobility has not been maintained.
6. Ischaemic contractures due to arterial damage. They may involve long muscles of forearm or small muscles of hand.
7. Painful conditions.

## Loss or decrease of movement, or alteration in movement patterns

This may be due to:
1. Angulation and rotation of bones following fractures which may cause the tendons to operate ineffectively. There may be apparent loss of joint control when an angled fracture is close to a joint, e.g. a fracture of the metacarpal neck, if not correctly aligned, can appear as loss of full extension of the metacarpophalangeal joint.
2. Paralysis of muscles due to a nerve lesion can produce an imbalance of movement, with resultant deformity. Trick movements may also be discovered. A muscle flicker or very weak contraction may indicate nerve regeneration. Stiff joints may make muscle testing difficult.
3. Muscle contracture due to ischaemia.

## Sensory changes

These will give an indication of the stage of nerve degeneration or regeneration.
1. Anaesthesia will result from an axonotmesis or neurotmesis and very temporarily from a neurapraxia also.
2. Hyperaesthesia is the first sensation experienced when some nerve regeneration has occurred. The 'pins and needles' feeling is due to the lack of insulation afforded by the myelin at this early recovery stage.
3. Hypoaesthesia follows the hyperaesthesia. Maturation of the myelin occurs, causing disappearance of the hyperaesthesia. The reduced or woolly sensation is due to the fact that some of the axons have been unable to regenerate to their correct end organs. This inevitably reduces the final degree of sensory recovery.
4. Hyperpathia, an extremely painful response to touch, may sometimes occur following nerve lesions.
5. The advance of the Tinel test suggests sensory nerve regeneration. It is accurate in a large proportion of patients with peripheral nerve damage, but is not totally infallible.

## Autonomic changes of the skin and nails

The changes that can be observed and palpated may accompany the previously mentioned motor and sensory changes and are the result of nerve involvement.

Skin changes include:
1. Loss of sweating which may be followed by excessive sweating.
2. Colour changes—purplish pink with loss of mottling.
3. Temperature takes on that of surroundings.
4. Scaly initially and shiny later.
5. Trophic lesions.
6. Ridges formed in nails.

Reflex sympathetic dystrophy must be considered if the above symptoms, combined with pain and swelling, present without direct nerve damage.

## DIFFERENTIATION BETWEEN JOINT STIFFNESS AND TETHERING OF TENDONS

It is particularly important to decide whether either or both stiffness and tethering may be preventing full movement.

*N.B.* Deformities do not necessarily limit function. This should be remembered when planning both conservative and surgical treatment. A very mobile and flail joint may also prove to be less functional than a stiff one, and a slightly contracted muscle may provide a useful tenodesis effect.

## TREATMENT PLANNING

An adequate programme should be arranged which will essentially:
1. Reduce oedema.
2. Treat pain.
3. Improve function mainly by mobilising joints, exercising and re-educating muscles, and re-educating sensation. Functional activities should play an ever-increasing role.
4. Attend to psychological, social and employment needs.

The problems as seen by the physiotherapist and other members of the team should be numbered, preferably in the order of priority. The initial treatment plan can then be drawn up and a programme arranged.

Intensive early treatment over a short period is far more effective than sporadic treatment for a much longer time span. This must be taken into account when planning the treatment programme. Full-time rehabilitation may make all the difference between a poor result and an efficiently functioning hand.

## REFERENCES

American Academy of Orthopaedic Surgery 1982 Joint motion—a method of measuring and recording. Churchill Livingstone, Edinburgh.

Bromley A I 1978 The patient care audit. Physiotherapy 64:9

Dellon A L 1984 Touch sensibility in the hand. Journal of Hand Surgery 9–B: 1

Heath J R 1978 Problem orientated medical systems. Physiotherapy 64: 9

Henderson W R 1948 Clinical assessment of peripheral nerve injuries: Tinel's test. Lancet 2: 801

Kaltenborn F M 1980 Mobilisation of the extremity joints. Olaf Norlis, Oslo

Maitland G D 1977 Peripheral manipulation. Butterworths, London

Medical Research Council 1981 Aids to the examination of the peripheral nervous system. HMSO, London

Richardson J A 1979 Problem orientated medical records and patient care audits in North America. Physiotherapy 65: 6

Wynn Parry C B 1981 Rehabilitation of the hand. Butterworths, London

## FURTHER READING

Anderson W F, Cowan N R 1966 Hand grip pressure in older people. British Journal of Preventive and Social Medicine 20: 141–147

Cantrell E G 1976 Measurement of weakness and dysfunction in the rheumatoid hand. Rheumatology and Rehabilitation 15(3)

Fernando M U, Robertson J C 1982 Grip strength in the healthy. Rheumatology and Rehabilitation 21: 179–181

Lister G 1984 The hand: diagnosis and implications, 2nd edn. Churchill Livingstone, Edinburgh

Reikeras O 1983 Bilateral differences of normal hand strength. Archives of Orthopaedic and Traumatic Surgery 101: 223–224

Wright V 1959 Some observations on diurnal variation of grip. Clinical Science 18: 17–23

# 3

# Physiotherapy management

It is essential that a physiotherapist is involved in the management of hand injuries to achieve the best results. The majority of patients following injury and surgery do not know either what or how much they should do with their hands. Moreover, even when well motivated, they will probably not have the suitable means with which to work at home.

In the past it was occasionally suggested that hand patients did not need formal treatment but that they should be sufficiently able to treat themselves. Experience has shown this to be totally incorrect and that all patients with hand injuries benefit from skilled treatment, be it sometimes very little. Expert advice and supervision may be adequate for some, while others may need extensive treatment; it is not always apparent which category each patient will fall into when he is first assessed.

All injuries, however minor, are entitled to this early assessment and treatment, and after the treatment ceases each patient should be reviewed to ensure that his progress has been maintained. One essential factor in achieving consistently good results is a dedicated team. This must include a skilled surgeon, experienced therapists, a social worker to provide support and of the utmost importance, a well-motivated patient. The value of having this team approach cannot be over-emphasised as it benefits everyone, especially the patient.

Clinics should be held every week if possible and all the therapists and the social worker should attend. The progress that the patient has made and any difficulty that has arisen should be discussed so that each member of the team will be aware of activity in other departments. In this way it can be ensured that all aspects of the patient's needs are covered. The resettlement officer should be involved early after injury, especially if the patient is likely to have difficulty at work. Advice from a clinical psychologist should be available if necessary.

A severe hand injury may well have a devastating effect on the life of the patient. For successful overall care the emotional, psychological and social needs of the patient should be handled sympathetically and with urgency. The physiotherapist plays an important role in listening to the patient's worries, providing reassurance, and communicating with the social worker or psychologist when necessary. As the patient spends more time with the therapist than most other members of the team a confidential relationship is likely to develop.

Providing adequate treatment for hand injuries should have high priority in all physiotherapy departments. Intensive early treatment over a short period is found to be far more effective than sporadic treatment for a longer time span. This must be taken into account when the treatment programme is planned. Full-time rehabilitation may make all the difference between a poor result and an efficiently functioning hand. A large proportion of severe hand injuries happen to people of working age, and their needs, both in getting them back to work and in looking after their leisure interests, should take precedence over some of the more chronic work of the department.

Patients with wrist and hand injuries are frequently treated in a group environment because of the large numbers involved. This plays an important role in treatment as the patient meets and works with others who have similar problems. However, every patient should be assessed separately and given individual treatment initially. This must be accompanied by a thorough explanation of the injury, the treatment to be given and the progress expected. Following this patients should be seen individually for a few minutes at least at every attendance of their class therapy.

Each patient must be able to demonstrate that he remembers his home exercises and is practising them. The measurements must also show that satisfactory progress is being maintained. Any problems such as pain and residual joint stiffness should be attended to urgently and individually. Even though patient numbers may be extremely high, as, for example, during a period of icy conditions in winter, these acute injuries must be treated adequately. With a hand injury to manage the physiotherapist must never put off until tomorrow the problems which need treatment today. This will inevitably produce disappointing results.

The physiotherapist's use of her own hands to make contact with the patient's injured one is extremely important. Not only can the difficulties be assessed by the 'feel' of the damaged hand, but the treatment can also be minutely adjusted according to the stage reached. Hand to hand contact is the most natural occurrence in our lives from infancy onwards, and it has the effect of reassuring the patient and helping him to regain confidence. This is partly because he is aware that the physiotherapist can experience and treat some of the problems with her finger tips, but also because she is willing to touch a hand which to him may still look unsightly. It may mean that the physiotherapist must wear gown, mask and gloves immediately following a severe injury in order to maintain aseptic conditions.

Management of hand injuries must progress continually and steadily through the various stages of injury, i.e. operation, healing and rehabilitation, in order to gain a maximum result. There is a gradual progression between the first and last stages, which are described in the following pages.

The stage at which energetic rehabilitation may commence depends very much on the degree of injury received, the surgery which has had to be performed, the healing achieved and the progress made. The time lapse before certain treatments may be safely given is only a rough estimate. Definite timings must be agreed upon between surgeon and therapist so that maximum effect is achieved and damage is not caused by starting treatment too soon.

Returning function to the hand is the most important aim of treatment and this must be remembered from the earliest treatment through to the final stages of rehabilitation. To achieve this end the reduction of oedema and pain must be tackled instantly, but the essential of all therapy is to retain the maximum range of joints.

## TREATMENT IN THE EARLY STAGES FOLLOWING INJURY AND OPERATION

Injury of the soft tissues inevitably results in cellular damage. An inflammatory process occurs which is followed about five days later by the commencement of healing and repair. Although repair cannot be hastened, certain factors assist and others will retard this healing process (Evans 1980). The timing of these stages must therefore be carefully observed. If too energetic treatment is given in the early stages it may exacerbate a greater inflammatory reaction which will result in the production of extensive fibrosis.

Following surgery, 3 weeks rest may be necessary before exercises to the injured part may commence. Physiotherapy can, however, be most influential during the early management of a hand injury, particularly in preventing or reducing any oedema. Any part of the upper limb or hand that is not immobilised must also be treated during this time, which will give patient and therapist the opportunity of getting to know one another.

### ASSESSMENT

Few of the assessments, as described in the previous chapter, can be performed at this early stage. Careful observation of the hand, its position, swelling and colour and the amount of movement, should therefore be made and recorded in the SOAP notes. Measurements should be taken of joints that are not immobilised, and sensation should be checked carefully for the first few days to ensure that bandages and plasters are not too tight. This could otherwise lead to the development of a neuropraxia.

### GENERAL TREATMENT

Attention should be paid to the patient's chest function following surgery, and the unaffected joints of the upper limb must be kept mobile. The shoulder in particular is liable to stiffen if not exercised, especially in elderly people. General fitness of the patient must also be considered early after injury and operation.

### Elevation

Elevation helps to lower the pressure in blood vessels, and aids lymphatic drainage of the exudate. This decrease of tissue pressure will automatically help to reduce the pain, which can be intense with a severely oedematous hand.

The hand should be supported in an elevated position both when the patient is in bed and when ambulant.

*In bed* the whole arm should be elevated, using a roller towel suspended from a drip stand. The edges of the towel are pinned together to prevent the hand from slipping out. The angle of the elbow should not be too acute, as this might restrict the drainage. Pillows should therefore be used to support the upper arm comfortably.

If the patient is discharged early and elevation at night is still essential a broom handle can be utilised when no stand is available. The broom, head upwards, can be fixed to the bed by a relatively simple attachment and a towel suspended from the broom head by the method already described. An alternative is to rest the arm on a large pile of pillows.

*When ambulant* the hand should be supported either in a Chessington type sling (Fig. 3.1a & b) (Wynn Parry 1981) or in a continuous strap sling (Fig. 3.2). Alternatively a high triangular sling can be used, but whichever method is chosen the hand should be held higher than the elbow, and the angle of the elbow should not be too acute.

### Cooling

A vasoconstriction of capillaries will help to prevent excess exudate. Cooling can be produced by use of a fan, or by applying towels (which have been wrung out in very cold water) to available skin. Ice packs should not be used in the first few days as they could produce a local vasodilatation which is undesirable as it could exacerbate the oedema.

### Pressure

Gentle massage may be given to reduce the exudate where undamaged skin is accessible. Care should be taken not to traumatise the tissues any further by pressing too deeply with the fingers.

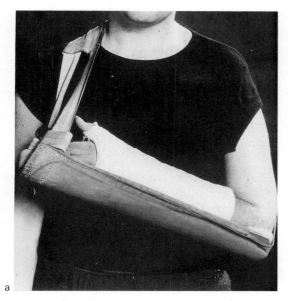
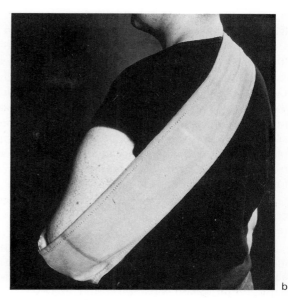

**Fig. 3.1(a & b)** The Chessington sling provides comfortable support with the weight taken over the unaffected shoulder. It is adjusted to increase the amount of hand elevation. This patient suffered multiple injuries to the upper limb.

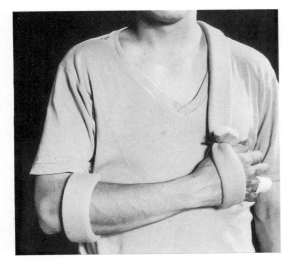

**Fig. 3.2** The continuous strap sling is a progression from the Chessington sling.

Closed environmental therapy (CET) may have been selected for the patient by the surgeon. This involves elevating the whole hand and forearm inside a plastic bag into which sterile air is blown at above normal atmospheric pressure. It enables movements to be carried out by the patient with his hand still in the bag.

## Movement

Gentle muscle contractions should be performed as soon as possible as they are one of the best means of assisting both venous and lymphatic drainage, and will not aggravate the inflammatory process. On approximately the fifth day, when the healing and repair stage has commenced, very gentle active movements should be given which will give a natural stretch to the damaged tissues. This movement is necessary to ensure that the collagen which is forming is laid down in an efficient linear structure. Fibrous tissue continues to contract for at least six months after healing, and will need repetitive active stretching for this length of time.

The initial exercises given can include isometric contractions and isotonic contractions through a small range. The range of movement is increased as the condition of the hand improves.

Even though the hand may be totally covered in dressings and splints, isometric muscle contractions can still be given when suitable. The unaffected part of the body must also be exercised immediately after injury.

Silicone oil has been found to be a suitable medium in which to carry out the early movement and muscle contractions, especially after crush and open injuries. The sterile oil is kept in a jar of sufficient size so that the whole hand may be immersed. Gentle exercises are performed, the patients like the feel of movement in this bland medium and healing appears to be accelerated (Gifford 1974). Debris from the injury will fall away and settle in the bottom of the jar and it may be left until the patient no longer requires this form of exercise. The silicone oil can then be cleaned and sterilised, or otherwise thrown away. It must not be used for other patients because of the likelihood of cross-infection. One great disadvantage is the high cost of the oil.

*Caution.* These early exercises must not involve contraction of muscles and tendons which have recently been repaired.

The active movements and contractions which may be given are listed below. All may not be suitable, however, so each individual patient's needs must be considered separately and carefully.

1. Wrist extension, flexion, radial and ulnar deviation.
2. Pronation and supination.
3. Flexion of all metacarpophalangeal and interphalangeal joints.
4. Extension of those joints.
5. Flexion of metacarpophalangeal joints together with extension of interphalangeal joints.
6. Flexion of interphalangeal joints together with extension of metacarpophalangeal joints.
7. Adduction of fingers and thumb followed by abduction of fingers and radial abduction of thumb.
8. Palmar abduction and adduction of thumb.
9. Opposition of thumb and little finger towards one another.
10. Flexion of thumb across palm followed by extension.

As has already been stressed, these active movements and contractions must be introduced with extreme care in order to improve the quality of healing. Very early passive movement and energetic exercises are contraindicated because they will only increase the inflammatory process and thus exacerbate the degree of fibrosis.

*Movement must never be given* if it is likely to jeopardise the results of surgery.

## Pulsed electro-magnetic fields (PEMF)

Early treatment with high frequency pulsed diathermy is advocated to reduce oedema and limit the degree of fibrous tissue formation (Barclay et al 1983). The quality of healing, particularly in the regeneration of nerves, is thereby accelerated and improved (Wilson & Jagerdeesh 1976, Raji & Bowden 1983). A higher dosage than for continuous diathermy may be given as the healing effect of pulsed current is minimal.

## Ultrasound

Early use of ultrasonics has been recommended for improving the quality of fibrous tissue repair, probably by the streaming of the collagen fibres (Dyson & Suckling 1978, Patrick 1978). A pulsed, low dose treatment should be used.

### Contraindications

The immediate area surrounding sutured tendons should not be treated with ultrasound post-operatively for 4 weeks at least as this has been shown to delay and even prevent healing (Roberts et al 1982).

## REHABILITATION STAGE

Physiotherapy is concerned with the restoration of normal function, which involves a combination of motor and sensory performance. The major part of treatment should therefore utilise movement whenever possible, facilitated maximally by the correct sensory input.

The physiotherapist should handle the injured hand frequently as this establishes a direct contact which is a normal part of life and is therefore of physical and psychological advantage. Much can be learnt by the therapist from the 'feel' of the hand, and the patient is reassured that his problems are better understood.

The principles of treatment, both post-operative or following injury, must be understood by the therapists so that they may develop a good working relationship with the surgeon in charge of the case. Case conferences should be held weekly to discuss the progress or any problems which may have arisen.

The patient himself must also feel involved both in the conference and in his treatment as it is the recovery of his hand that is at stake. A description should be given to him of his injury, the surgical procedures which may have been performed, and the probable length of time before some normal function will return. It is preferable that he understands the process of recovery, such as the effects following nerve degeneration. This will stop him from becoming too depressed while he watches any wasting and deformity worsen.

Good motivation is essential for the best possible recovery in hand function. The patient who accepts his injury and is determined to improve as quickly as possible will achieve far better results than he who indulges in recriminations and nurses his hand protectively. Delay in receiving compensation is likely to reduce some patients' motivation considerably.

Surgical procedures will have been performed on most severe injuries during the first few weeks and stitches are usually removed between 10 to 14 days post-operatively. Physiotherapy should already have been commenced by this stage.

The patient is usually ready for an increase in his treatment regime three to four weeks after surgery or injury. The hand, with its many joints, stiffens remarkably quickly, especially following gross oedema, and time must not be lost in recovering movement. Joints that are immobilised for 6 weeks or more are liable to become permanently stiff and the soft tissues will lose their elasticity.

Assessments as described in the previous chapter should now be carried out. They enable the problems to be identified and form a base for evaluating progress. Measurements are important as they make it easier for the patient and physiotherapist to see improvements. A few degrees of change in each joint each week is perfectly satisfactory, but is difficult to recognise without accurate measurement. The patient will be looking at his hand all day and every day, and he will be pleasantly surprised to see this improvement recorded on his flow chart.

Treatments given must be realistic in intensity and full time rehabilitation should be available for the patient with severe injuries. This will achieve a more effective return to normality than only one treatment session given daily. An early recovery and return to work makes economic sense besides being of tremendous psychological value to the patient.

## Planning treatment

Priorities may be difficult to select in a severe injury when there are many problems to treat. It must be remembered that the hand is a functioning mechanism, and methods for reduction of oedema, relief of pain and mobilising of joints are all a preparation for exercise therapy and functional rehabilitation. The initial programme should be arranged with the mutual agreement of all therapists. Any change in priorities should be discussed at the weekly case conference and the necessary alterations be made to the programme.

The treatments which follow are in the approximate order in which a session should normally progress. The priorities do not necessarily follow in the same order.
1. Preparation and warm-up
2. Oedema reduction
3. Pain reduction
4. Skin and nail care
5. Scars and soft tissue care
6. Joint movement
7. Muscle activity
8. Functional movements.
Teaching, advice and counselling should continue throughout.

The techniques of treatment given will frequently be effective for more than one of the aims. For example, active exercises will reduce oedema, reduce pain and improve both joint movement and muscle function. Overlapping will therefore be inevitable but at the same time beneficial. If pain is severe it is found that treatments given little and often are more effective and more acceptable to the patient than long sessions.

## Preparation for treatment

An introductory warm-up should, whenever possible, be given prior to any specific treatment. In a rehabilitation unit the standard procedure is for general but simple exercises to be performed to music at the start of the day. If this facility is not available the patient should exercise his hand for a few minutes in an arm bath of warm water, or saline if there are open areas.

A good circulation is essential for effective hand recovery and a warm glove or mitt must therefore be worn during cold weather. A simple form of mitt can be made by cutting off 25 cm of a discarded sweater or track suit sleeve and stitching it up with a rounded end. Some hands and fingers are so contracted that they are difficult to get into an ordinary glove, while a mitt is easy to slip on.

## OEDEMA

Oedema, with the resultant increase of pressure in the tissues, reduces movement, causes pain, and if untreated develops into fibrous tissue. All possible means must be utilised to reduce it quickly and efficiently. This includes elevation, mechanical pressure methods and, most effective of all, the patient's own activity. An explanation must be given to the patient as to why this is so important.

*Elevation* should be continued both when the patient is in bed at night and during the day, as described on p. 62.

During treatment the hand and arm are easily elevated by resting them on pillows against the raised back-rest of a plinth (Fig. 3.3). All treatments such as massage, joint movements and exercises should be carried out in this position.

*Ice baths* using a mulch of ice and water help to reduce oedema by causing a vasoconstriction of the capillaries (Fig. 3.4). The hand can be moved in the ice and the patient should attempt first to make a fist and then to extend his fingers. Two or three minutes are found adequate and if it becomes very uncomfortable the hand can be taken out and

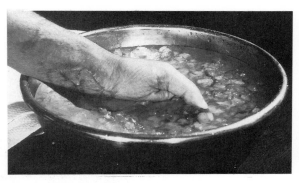

**Fig. 3.4** Ice baths, using a mulch of ice and water, for reducing oedema.

dried before re-immersing. Although it is not very pleasant patients adjust remarkably quickly to this treatment and report that their hand feels more mobile afterwards. If ice packs are used care must be taken not to produce an undesirable vasodilatation.

A small area can be treated locally by using an ice cube or compressed crushed ice and rubbing it over the affected area for a minute or two. Another option is to give contrast baths, which alternately produce a vasoconstriction followed by a vasodilation, thus improving the circulation generally.

Ice is contraindicated for a peripheral nerve lesion with its associated autonomic disturbance, as the part will become very cold and take some time to warm.

The above methods have been found more suitable than wax baths. The heat tends to make the hand swell and is a passive type of treatment. The temperature of the wax also needs to be lowered or burns may occur due to the lack of circulatory response associated with nerve lesions.

*Pneumotherapy* may be given in the physiotherapy department, and two methods are available. The first is pulsed environmental therapy (PET), with the arm placed inside a single layer bag and pressurised air blown in around the hand. A separate bag must be kept for each patient when using PET in order to avoid cross infection. The second is a technique with the arm placed inside a double layer plastic sleeve. Air is blown between the layers and also between the plastic and the skin. Care must be taken to ensure that the finger

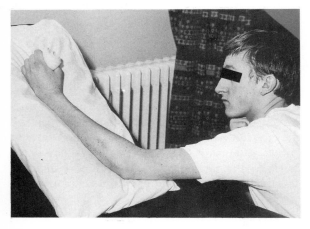

**Fig. 3.3** The arm and hand are easily elevated during treatment by resting against the raised back-rest of a plinth.

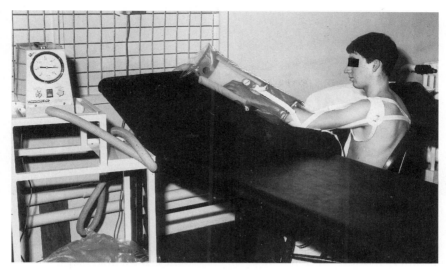

**Fig. 3.5** Reducing oedema by pneumotherapy, with the arm in elevation.

tips do not protrude beyond the end of the sleeve, and that folds of plastic are never allowed to traumatise the skin. The arm should always be placed in slight elevation for both these methods.

Use of these pneumotherapy techniques allows the therapist to carry on with treatment of other patients while the oedema is being reduced.

*Massage in elevation* using effleurage and gentle kneading, especially for small areas such as web spaces, will disperse oedema efficiently. The physiotherapist must be careful not to traumatise delicate skin and scar tissue by using too deep a pressure of the finger tips. Massage can be time consuming and is not always found to be the most cost- or time-effective treatment for large areas of oedema.

*Exercises in elevation*, both active and passive, can be performed with the patient's arm resting against the raised back-rest of a plinth (Fig. 3.3). Non-specific exercises, i.e. squeezing a ball or grip, making a fist followed by extending the fingers, and circumducting the hand at the wrist, can be performed by the patient while he is waiting for the physiotherapist's attention.

*Rubber bandaging* of the fingers can help to disperse oedema. A rubber strip approximately 40 cm x 2 cm is wound firmly on to the finger, commencing at the tip and working proximally (Fig. 3.6). Immediately it reaches the base of the finger the rubber is unwound and the procedure repeated.

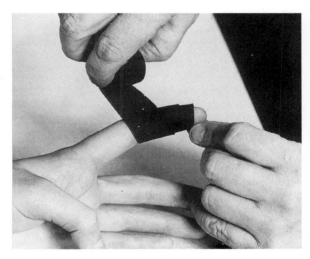

**Fig. 3.6** Oedema of the finger can be reduced by bandaging from distal to proximal with a rubber strip.

This should be carried out several times for each finger. As the oedema is reduced a greater stretch can be put on the rubber as it is bandaged around.

This method can also be used for gross oedema of the carpometacarpal area, but is not as effective as for the fingers. The hollow of the palm will need to be padded, and a wider rubber strip used.

*Finger stalls* can be made from elasticated material such as double thickness Tubigrip which is stitched to form a double finger stall (Fig. 3.7a & b).

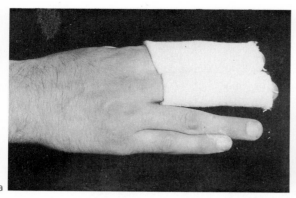
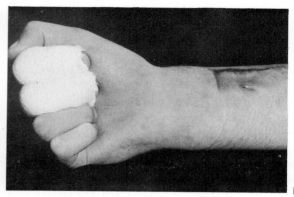

**Fig. 3.7(a & b)**   Double thickness Tubigrip makes an effective double fingerstall which helps to prevent oedema from returning.

It should be pulled down firmly on to the fingers. Two double stalls can be used if all four fingers are swollen. This technique is effective in preventing the return of oedema after its reduction by the methods previously described.

Elasticated gloves are available commercially and can be useful for preventing the return of whole hand oedema, but because pressure is not exerted by the glove on the palm it cannot be totally effective. Covering the finger tips also reduces sensation and therefore the functional use of the hand, so that a glove with just the tips free should be selected.

*Interferential treatment* has been found to assist the dispersal of areas of persistent oedema. Its effect must be monitored carefully, especially when there are autonomic problems.

## PAIN

Pain is a complex phenomenon which is influenced by factors such as the type and severity of injury, the inhibitory mechanisms, any neurogenic responses and the temperament of the patient. It results from increased central excitation of the injury detection cells in the dorsal horn. This excitation is effected by the discharges, mainly from the nociceptors and the high threshold, small diameter afferent fibres.

It is known that the central excitation is inhibited by the discharges of low threshold afferents and that it is under powerful control by the systems descending from the brain into the spinal cord (Wall 1985). This means that by stimulating the mechanoreceptors and by occupying the patient with interesting activities pain can be considerably diminished. The age-old method of a mother whose child has hurt himself, is to rub and kiss the part better and give a sweet to distract him, thus increasing both peripheral and central inhibition. It is important that these principles are also applied by the therapist when attempting to relieve pain.

The cause of the pain must be treated initially as well as the pain itself. Injury and operations will inevitably produce pain and they may also produce oedema, which when severe can be an extremely distressful condition. The oedema must be reduced quickly both for reasons of distress and for its fibrotic effect.

It is vital that pain is treated immediately it is experienced; otherwise it might become 'programmed' into the patient's life. Even when the cause has been removed the pain will sometimes remain. Most therapists will have treated patients who fit into this category. Pain should never be belittled or disbelieved. To the patient it is a very real and unpleasant actuality. It may be his main or only problem, especially if it has not been treated until late, and will need urgent attention.

Pain can be classified in various ways, such as primary and secondary, acute and chronic. The physiotherapist who treats hand injuries will recognise pain which can be divided into three main categories. Fortunately the majority of hand patients will only experience the first.

1. Primary or acute pain.
2. Residual pain.
3. Chronic pain.

## Primary or acute pain

All patients will suffer pain following injury and surgery: it is a normal response. It should be treated with pain-killing drugs and will usually be gone within 2–3 weeks. Physiotherapy which reduces oedema and therefore relieves pain should be introduced immediately.

Primary pain may also be experienced when treatment techniques such as passive stretching are carried out in later stages by the physiotherapist. The stretch is of relatively short duration and when released the pain should cease almost instantly. Most patients can understand this rationale and are usually well prepared to tolerate this short-term discomfort.

## Residual pain

Pain may remain after 3 to 4 weeks when it becomes classified as secondary pain. It is usually due to lengthy immobilisation, lack of normal activity and very often too little therapy, thereby leaving some residual oedema.

The introduction of intensive treatment, with a regime as energetic as is suitable, will usually have a quick and beneficial effect. Physiotherapy techniques should be designed not only to treat any residual problems such as oedema but to activate the inhibitory mechanisms, thereby reducing pain. When this occurs the patient should be able to use his limb more freely.

## Chronic pain

Pain which persists for several weeks after injury and is severe and intractable is secondary pain, but it is a comparatively rare condition. Approximately only 5% of patients with nerve injury experience causalgia, and relatively few patients actually develop reflex sympathetic dystrophy. This latter condition is more likely to follow a minor injury such as a sprain, a Colles fracture or soft tissue surgery, especially when little early formal treatment has been given. Sympathetic disorder,

with lack of both central and peripheral inhibition, is largely responsible for this painful state.

Intensive treatment must be given for the pain, combined with functional rehabilitation whenever possible, in a determined attempt to solve a difficult problem. If it is unresponsive to treatment, referral to a pain clinic may be necessary. There may be both pathological and psychological factors involved (Lipton 1979).

## Physiotherapy treatment

The initial cause of pain must be established so that it can be treated correctly. There may have been soft tissue damage, oedema, and loss of mobility, all of which should be quickly improved by physiotherapy techniques. Ice, heat and exercise, the use of TNS, PEMF, interferential treatment and the vibrator have all been found to provide some relief particularly by those patients with the first two categories of pain. Acupuncture should be considered as an alternative treatment when other methods fail.

As much sensory in-put and as normal a movement as possible will produce stimulation of the mechanoreceptors via the large diameter low threshold fibres. This probably closes the gate to the pain-carrying small unmyelinated C-fibres, as described in the 'gate-control' theory of pain (Melzack & Wall 1965). The addition of an interesting occupation in order to provide distraction is the best means in helping to diminish the pain.

Care must be taken not to worsen the pain of an already painful hand by increasing the discharges from the nociceptors. All treatments must be gentle at first and increase in intensity gradually when it is seen that no adverse effect results.

TNS is a cheap and efficient means for stimulating the large diameter afferents. The stimulator is small, easily used at home by the patient and safely worn for several hours at a time. (Most other pain-relieving methods used by physiotherapists have only a short duration effect). The electrodes are easily fixed to the skin and the battery operated stimulator can be pocketed so that the treatment may be used for as long as the patient desires. There appear to be very few undesirable effects.

Stimulators that can be switched from the higher frequency of 10–100 Hz to the lower 0–10 Hz are particularly useful. The higher frequency should be used first, thereby utilising the pain-gate theory, and once some relief has been gained the stimulator can be switched to the lower frequency. It is thought likely that the lower frequency effects the release of endogenous opiates and endorphins, thus helping to relieve the pain.

### Electrode positioning in TNS

There are no set rules for electrode placement and some days of trial are probably needed to discover the best position (Frampton 1981). A dual output stimulator which allows two sets of electrodes to be used on the lower part of the forearm, has been found effective for treating widely distributed pain in the hand.

As a guide for positioning, the electrodes should be:

1. On skin with sensation. This is absolutely essential.
2. On either side, or distal and proximal, but not immediately over the painful area.
3. Proximal to painful area in hand, over applicable nerve supply.
4. On both anterior and posterior aspects of forearm when the whole hand is painful, using two sets of electrodes.
5. Over acupuncture points and channels (Lewith 1980).

### Application

The patient should record the level of pain on his pain chart both before and after treatment in order to judge effectiveness. He should be instructed on the use of the stimulator so that he can adjust it for himself, and use it at home if necessary.

The malleable electrodes, spread with gel for good conductivity, are attached to the skin using Micropore tape (Fig. 3.8a & b). Occasionally they are also bandaged to retain good contact while the hand is being used. Self-adhesive electrodes are available for patients who have difficulty in attaching electrodes.

The current is turned on and increased gradually until the patient feels that a comfortable degree has been reached. he adjusts the rate to his liking, and increases the pulse width (if this adjustment is available). When utilising the gate control theory, which is usual for the start of treatment, the patient is likely to benefit by a fairly strong sensation of current, but it must never be painful as this might increase the discharges from the nociceptors.

The stimulator should be left on for at least two hours when experimenting for correct placement, and for 6–8 hours to give any real benefit. Amount of current, time it is on and position of electrodes should be adjusted until the best result is achieved. If no effect has been found during the first two weeks it is unlikely to become a useful treatment.

At the end of treatment the position of the electrodes is recorded and the pain relief charted. The next day it is important to discover the duration of any relief.

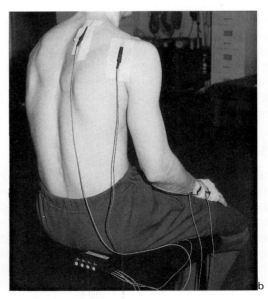

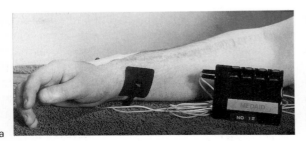

**Fig. 3.8** TNS can be used to relieve pain. (a) Locally, through and through the wrist joint. (b) When pain radiates down the arm into the TI distribution.

TNS can also be valuable while the physio-therapist is giving an uncomfortable treatment. Sometimes even the lightest touch is painful and this can be reduced considerably by TNS in the majority of cases, allowing mobilising, stretch techniques and tapping of painful neuromata to be performed. Use of TNS with pain caused by nerve lesions and reflex sympathetic dystrophy will be discussed in a later chapter.

*Precautions*

1. Electrodes should not be placed over broken skin.
2. TNS must not be used by patients with pace-makers.
3. It should only be used during pregnancy or for patients with heart disease when prescribed by a physician.
4. Patients should be cautioned not to exacerbate a painful condition by over-exercising during the pain relief.
5. A few patients may be allergic to the gel, the tape or even the current.

**Guanethidine blocks**

If the pain is intractable the physician may pre-scribe guanethidine which produces sympathetic blocking. The guanethidine is injected and, if effective in pain relief, must be followed immedi-ately by exercising and occupation with functional activities. The procedure may need to be repeated several times to have a cumulative effect.

SKIN CARE

Following either injury or operation the skin will become dry and scaly (Fig. 3.9) but this can be improved quickly by the physiotherapist's treat-ment. An arm bath of warm water, or saline if there are residual open areas, will help to soften the dried skin. The hand should be exercised in the water for three or four minutes as has been de-scribed in the general preparation. While it is being dried, much of the softened dead skin can be gently removed. The application of a hydrous ointment will assist in improving the skin condition.

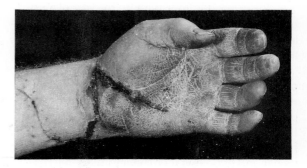

**Fig. 3.9** Following injury and operation the skin will become dry and scaly.

Nails should be cut by the physiotherapist when necessary and the nail beds attended to. It is im-portant that the patient does not damage himself with scissors, and as he will probably be unable to cut the nails of his other hand he will need this attention also.

This is a good moment to advise the patient about any anaesthetic areas and the danger of burns. Burns with resulting blisters can be caused by a variety of means and patients have to be re-minded frequently to watch what they are doing if they are near or using anything hot. The author has experienced patients burning themselves on radi-ators, kettles and teapots; by letting a little finger slip down on to the iron being used; by picking up a hot potato for peeling and by a lighted cigarette burning across anaesthetic fingers. Cold burns and friction can also blister the skin.

Blisters, if they do arise, should not be pricked but should be left uncovered, unless they are likely to be damaged. If they burst they should be dressed to keep them clean. A lesion of this type will usually take much longer to heal because of the poor nu-trition of the area.

CIRCULATION AND SOFT TISSUES

It is imperative that an adequate circulation is maintained to encourage healing and regeneration. A warm glove or mitt must be worn in cold weather to keep the hand warm, particularly for those patients with nerve involvement.

If an artery has been ligated, the circulation will be reduced considerably. The collateral supply can, however, be improved by the use of contrast baths. The effect of alternate vasoconstriction followed by vasodilatation of the capillaries will help to increase the blood flow in the affected area.

Attention should be paid to the soft tissues to prevent loss of suppleness and contracture of the web spaces. Daily stretching of the webs and a passive mobilising of the hand when active movement is absent will help to retain mobility. The physiotherapist should stretch the tissues of the thenar and hypothenar eminences by firmly running her hands over the skin, and continue this stretch to the finger tips. By holding either side of the patient's hand with both hers she can flatten and fully arch the hand, and then move either side in a counterdirection.

Soft tissue injury to the forearm may cause considerable loss of movement in the hand. Vascular damage can produce Volkmann's ischaemic contracture or there may be a direct muscle injury. Both are likely to result in loss of the full contractile and extensile property of the muscles and the developing contracture will cause a loss of extension in the distal joints. In severe cases it can affect the extensors as well as the flexors. Injury at the level distal to the wrist, when ischaemia results, will produce contracture of the intrinsic muscles. Because they are so small, these muscles are particularly difficult to stretch once contracted. To stretch them maximally the interphalangeal joints should first be fully flexed and then the metacarpophalangeal joints extended (Fig. 3.10). Any

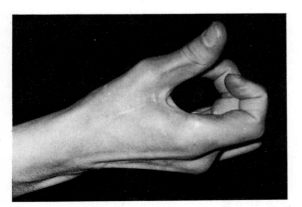

**Fig. 3.10** Attempted flexion of the interphalangeal joints together with extension of the metacarpophalangeal joints. Note that this is impossible for the middle finger because of an intrinsic contracture.

stretch splinting for an intrinsic contracture must attempt to achieve this position.

The soft tissues and webs which have already become contracted should be given a deep stretching type of kneading followed by gentle but firm passive stretching, active movements and stretch splinting. Very restricted web spaces will benefit from Polyform serial splinting, but if the circulation or sensation is impaired Plastazote is preferable (see p. 109).

## SCARS

Scars will need treatment especially if they are adherent and surrounded by hard indurated subcutaneous tissue. Ultrasonics is given early to help reduce and stream the collagen formation and soften the scar tissue (Dyson & Suckling 1978). Following healing, gentle massage should be given with a soft hydrous ointment around the scar. Too deep a massage directly over the scar in the early stages is likely to cause blistering.

As the scar tissue strengthens the massage should become deeper, the fingers or thumb being used to achieve some depth. Lanolin ointment is now found useful as it makes a tacky contact with the skin and prevents the sliding which occurs with hydrous ointment. If no medium at all is used the skin might be frictioned painfully. The whole surrounding area of induration should be massaged deeply as it has an efficient softening effect.

If the scar is adherent to tendons the freeing of this adherence must be attempted. Tension should be applied first in a caudad and then in a cephalad direction. The patient flexes his fingers to apply this tension while the scar is frictioned over the taut tendon (Fig. 3.11a & b). This is repeated in the opposite direction, usually by the therapist extending the fingers passively whilst stretching the adherent scar with deep frictional massage.

Exercises are then given to stretch these adherent structures (see p. 81). Strong resisted exercising is one of the best means by which these adhesions will be stretched and freed, and should be given at the earliest stage that is considered safe. Polyform splinting is found very effective in softening any scar and indurated tissue; at the same time it can provide a stretch.

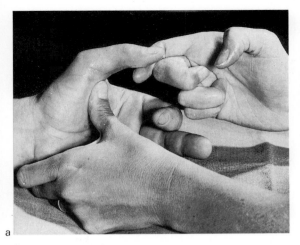
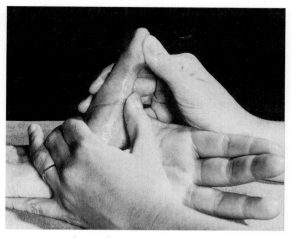

**Fig. 3.11** Frictional type massage being given across and around the adherent tendon of FPL. Tension is applied at the same time (a) by the patient's active contraction against slight resistance (b) by the physiotherapist.

Gross adherence of scarring can cause considerable reduction of functions, and when conservative treatment fails surgery may be necessary to free the adherent tissues. Physiotherapy should be commenced within the first 2–3 days following surgery to retain the movement gained.

## JOINT MOBILITY

A full range of pain-free movement is in most circumstances the aim of treatment for all joints of the hand. This involves the maintenance of the mobile joints or the mobilisation of those that have become stiff. The hand functions most essential to the patient should be ascertained so that the priorities for joint mobilisation can be decided. Before fully mobilising the joint it should be considered whether active control is likely to be regained or not, as a permanently flail joint could possibly prove to be a handicap. However, with the improved techniques of surgery, some function can usually be returned to mobile joints.

The most functional position of wrist, thumb and fingers, especially if there is residual stiffness, is found when contact can be made between tips of thumb, index and middle fingers. This happens to be in the close-packed range and has a bearing therefore on both the position of immobilisation and the direction in which the mobilisation will later be necessary.

### Position of immobilisation

As the joints are usually the major consideration, they should be immobilised in the close-packed position. The forearm should be in the mid-position, the wrist in some extension with ulnar deviation, the metacarpophalangeal joints in flexion and the interphalangeal joints in nearly full extension. The thumb should be abducted and rotated medially. Thus the ligaments are on a stretch, the capsules spiralised and the joint surfaces maximally congruent. The hand is now in a taut 'safe' position.

Rarely should the hand be immobilised in the extended position and never in either the fully flexed or claw position. Occasionally the position of function, with a small amount of interphalangeal joint flexion, is considered more desirable.

### Direction of mobilisation

When the hand has been immobilised in this 'safe' position the mobilisation is made easier as the direction of movement to be regained is into the loose-packed range. If, however, immobilisation has been in a loose-packed position the mobilisation must be into the close-packed range and the results are then frequently found to be disappointing.

### Priorities of joint movement

The extended, frozen hand which cannot flex is firstly of no practical use at all and secondly is very

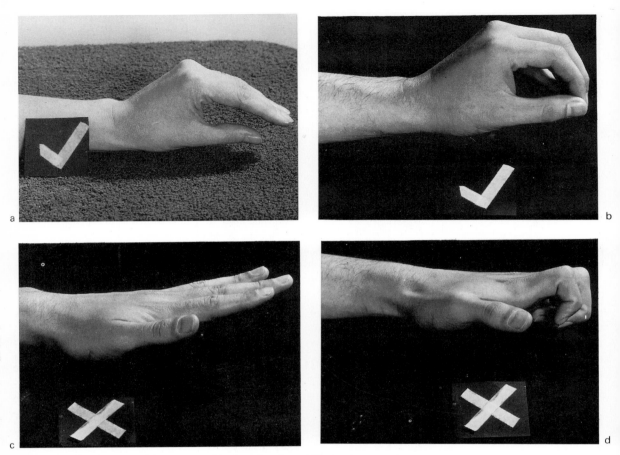

**Fig. 3.12(a–d)** Correct and incorrect positioning when immobilisation is essential.

difficult and time-consuming to mobilise. For every-day use it is important to improve the movements of grasp and thumb and finger approximation. When they have been nearly totally regained, attention should be switched to regaining full hand extension. If the finger movements are likely to remain limited it is the hand that recovers meta-carpophalangeal joint flexion which proves to be most functional.

The needs of the patient's employment and his leisure activities must be taken into consideration when deciding the priorities.

### Radio-ulnar joint

Pronation and supination are essential to increase the variety of functional movements. Immobilis-ation is normally in the mid-position, and the first

priority is to regain pronation, as it has slightly greater functional value than supination.

### Wrist joint

For most of the time the hand will function more effectively with the wrist in some degree of exten-sion. This enables the long flexors of the fingers to produce a stronger grasp than with the wrist in flexion. Flexion is utilised, however, when food is placed in the mouth with the fingers, so that eating is more difficult when wrist flexion is limited.

It is more important to regain ulnar deviation than radial deviation. Grasp of a knife, a hammer or an axe-handle needs some ulnar deviation in order to position the implement in the same align-ment as the forearm.

The priorities of wrist movement are therefore:

1. Wrist extension
2. Ulnar deviation
3. Wrist flexion
4. Radial deviation.

*Joints of the fingers*

The order of priority to regain digit function is as follows:
1. Metacarpophalangeal joint flexion
2. Interphalangeal joint extension
3. Metacarpophalangeal joint extension and interphalangeal joint flexion.

With so many joints in the fingers and so little distance between them it may be difficult to increase active metacarpophalangeal joint flexion and interphalangeal joint extension simultaneously. In this case it is simpler to improve firstly flexion and secondly extension of all joints together. Having achieved an increase in one direction, the therapist switches to the opposite direction, at the same time ensuring that there is no decrease of the initial gain. Flexion is always the first priority in order to attain the ability to grasp and also because stiff extended fingers can provide no function at all.

For mechanical reasons it is simpler in the later stages, when the therapist can use passive stretch and serial splinting techniques, to regain extension and more difficult to regain full active flexion. This is a further reason for improving flexion during the early treatment.

*Joints of the thumb*

Co-ordination between eye and thumb is a highly developed function which ensures the ability to grasp objects and pick up small items with accuracy. Correct positioning together with sufficient movement of the thumb will therefore need urgent consideration, as without either the hand may be severely handicapped.

Palmar abduction and medial rotation at the carpometacarpal joint must be adequate to enable the tips of the fingers to flex and approximate with the tip of the thumb. Limited range at either the interphalangeal or metacarpophalangeal joints, however, is not so very disabling, provided that there is some movement in one of these joints and that carpometacarpal joint movement is good.

The priorities of movement of the thumb are therefore:
1. Abduction of the carpometacarpal joint
2. Medial rotation at the same joint
3. Flexion and extension of the metacarpophalangeal joint
4. Flexion and extension of the interphalangeal joint.

## MOBILISING TECHNIQUES

Commencement of treatment should be early, but the timing must depend on the type and severity of the injury. The physiotherapist, having assessed the affected joints, should make use of all available information such as the diagnosis and the degree of bone, joint, tendon or nerve injury in order to select the most suitable technique for retaining or regaining joint mobility. The timing of activities should be agreed upon with the surgeon, such as when resistance may be added and passive stretch given. Some clarification of these times will be given in the next chapter. It must be remembered that frequently there are many complicating factors besides the stiff joint itself.

The techniques which can be used for joint mobilising include active, accessory and passive physiological movements, passive stretching and the use of orthoses.

### Active movements

Active movement, when available, should be used for both retaining and recovering range and for improving function. The patient's muscle power should be utilised as early as permitted in order to return the hand to normal use. The therapist can ensure that the patient actively stretches his joints and contracted tissues for himself by applying resistence but at the same time allowing movement into the fullest range possible.

Joints normally activated by the muscles which are now paralysed, are liable to stiffen rapidly unless their mobility is maintained passively. Conversely, they will mobilise more easily as soon as active movement returns. Efforts should therefore be made to re-educate and strengthen the muscle actively as quickly as possible.

Active exercise, including normal physiological movements of both individual and groups of muscles, patterns of movement as in PNF, and functional activities, should all be given to improve joint range.

*Contraindications for mobilising by active movements include:*

1. Immediately following severe injury (first 3–4 days)
2. Following nerve and tendon surgery (3 weeks)
3. Acute inflammatory joint disease
4. Recent nearby and unstable fractures
5. Resistance may need to be delayed after surgery.

## Accessory movements

These passive gliding movements should be graded for both stiffness and pain. The 0–4 scale (Maitland 1977) may be used to show the degree or lack of accessory movement (4 being full movement). On passive testing a certain motion may be identified as producing the same pain as with active functional movement. Frequently this is very localised and will respond quickly to treatment.

Most joints of the hand are mobilised by the distal part being moved on the proximal. The joint line and surfaces should be palpated and the proximal part supported firmly with one hand. The therapist uses her other hand to mobilise the joints, the distal part being moved in a gliding motion on the proximal. Small repetitive oscillations will usually increase range without causing pain, but a small amount of traction to the joint may make treatment more comfortable. Antero–posterior gliding movements should be given to all joints of the hand, with lateral gliding also at the metacarpophalangeal joints. The movements of the thumb are the same as in the fingers but with additional lateral gliding and rotation at the sellar joint and with a slight alteration in the planes of movement.

The mechanics of the joint influences the direction in which the accessory movement is performed. Joints which are concavo-convex (concave proximally and convex distally as in the radio-carpal joint) should have the distal part mobilised

on the proximal in a dorsal direction to improve flexion and in a volar direction to improve extension (Fig. 3.13a & b). Those joints which are convex-concave, i.e. the metacarpophalangeal and interphalangeal joints, should have the distal part mobilised on the proximal in a volar direction to improve flexion, and in a dorsal direction to improve extension (Fig. 3.13c & d). Accessory range will always be greatest with the joint loose-packed, and this is therefore the most desirable position in which to perform these techniques.

Slight rotation of the joints, which occurs in functional movements such as grasping a large object, should be reproduced, first with traction and then with approximation. The approximation may be found to produce the same pain as is experienced during function. Further mobilising of

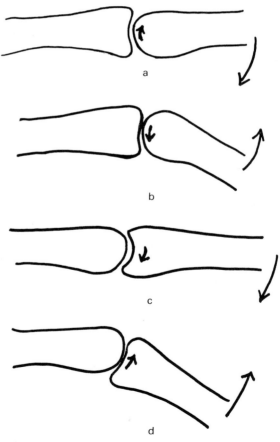

**Fig. 3.13** The direction of accessory movement, indicated by the small arrows, is influenced by the shape of the joint surfaces: (a) & (b) Concavo–convex (c) & (d) Convex–concave

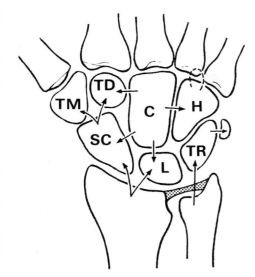

**Fig. 3.14**  Kaltenborn's ten movements of the wrist.

the joint with some traction will usually reduce this pain.

Limited space precludes the inclusion of detailed information on the treatment of each joint as this can be found elsewhere (Maitland 1977). The carpal region, however, deserves special mention. Following wrist injury or any lengthy immobilisation of the whole hand the wrist is frequently found to be very stiff, with loss of extension in particular. The many joints of the carpus are normally responsible for much of the wrist movement. If they lose the ability to glide on one another it is this decrease in movement, and the pain on movement, which may well be the cause of wrist stiffness.

For this reason the intercarpal joints should be examined and mobilised carefully. The capitate, which is aptly described as the keystone of the carpus (Kaltenborn 1980), should be identified first. Lying just proximal to the bases of the second and third metacarpals, it is easily palpated dorsally when the hand and wrist are flexed.

The other bones of the carpus are mobilised around the capitate (Fig. 3.14) with the wrist in flexion. All are then moved together on the radius and the ulnar styloid ligament.

*Contraindications to accessory movements include:*

1. An acutely inflamed joint
2. Any recent nearby fractures
3. Recent joint injuries.

**Passive physiological movement**

A normal joint without injury can safely be immobilised for 2 to 3 weeks before pathological changes occur. Over longer periods one or two movements a day are necessary to retain full mobility of an inactive joint.

This means that when muscles are paralysed but the joint is freely mobile the range can be maintained by giving passive physiological movements. The joint must be moved through the full range in all the directions that those muscles can normally achieve. The proximal part is supported firmly and the distal component is then moved through the full range available. The correct direction of the accessory movements must be incorporated at the same time (Fig. 3.13a, b, c & d).

If the joint is stiff through part of its range the free range must be maintained and any stiff extreme treated by small oscillations into that stiffness. Some distraction of the joint may help reduce any discomfort during movement.

**Combined passive physiological movements**

All the joints should be mobilised together in normal functional movements.

1. Press the metacarpophalangeal joints flat, and then into their arched position at the same time taking the thumb right across the palm.
2. The fingers should be rotated all together with some traction.
3. With the hand relaxed it can be shaken or tapped loosely on to a pillow, by holding it around the wrist.

*Contraindications to passive physiological movement include:*

1. Swollen and inflamed joints
2. Intracapsular damage
3. Recent direct joint injury
4. Nearby mobile fractures.

**Passive stretching**

If results from the previous treatments are slow, passive stretching may be considered, especially when the joint stiffness is combined with soft tissue injury and adherence. The technique should be similar to the passive physiological movements, applying the same direction of joint accessory movement. Strong active exercising should always follow passive stretching. This method should not be used if there is any articular surface injury, and never before 8 weeks have elapsed following nerve and tendon suture.

The therapist should support the proximal part firmly and stretch the distal component slowly and gradually into the stiff range (Fig. 3.15) applying slight traction at the same time. It should never be continued into a position which causes undue pain. The movements must be slow and sustained as this allows the therapist to watch the patient's face and to stop the stretch immediately it becomes painful. Fast and jerky movements might tear adhesions which would cause the release of further fibrinogen. The desired effect is to stretch any adhesions and contracted tissues slowly.

The tension of the stretch must also be released gradually, and the discomfort should then disappear rapidly. Any residual pain after a second or two indicates that too strong a stretch has been given. If the joint is painful or hot and swollen some hours following treatment it must be rested until this settles. The next treatment must give a minimal stretch and build up very gradually.

Patients may find this treatment uncomfortable, possibly painful, depending on the degree of stretch applied. Explanations must be given: most patients will understand the rationale and cope with this discomfort knowing that it will only last a short time and disappear as soon as the stretch is released. An extreme reaction to a very mild stretch may very occasionally occur and this can usually be reduced by the application of TNS prior to and during the stretch.

On-going assessments and measurements must be carried out if this treatment is to be used successfully. It is essential to be sure that it is having a corrective effect: it should not be left to guesswork.

If adherence and scarring are particularly dense and extensive, the passive stretch may eventually produce considerable discomfort in the joints. This is due to lack of extensability in the fibrous scar tissue, so that on application of stretch the joints are being compressed which in the end becomes painful. When this occurs, with no improvement evident when measured over one or two weeks, conservative treatment is unlikely to succeed. The patient should be referred to the surgeon who may consider releasing the adherent structures surgically at a suitable time.

*Contraindications to passive stretch include:*

1. Articular surface damage
2. Unstable, nearby fractures
3. Recent surgery of tendons and nerves (8–9 weeks)
4. Inflammatory disease affecting joints.

**Orthoses**

Having increased the passive range of a joint by the previously described techniques, splints can be used effectively and easily to maintain this increase. Any splint that is needed should be made by the physiotherapist who normally treats the patient, after the mobilising techniques have been applied.

If the treatment methods are producing extremely slow results splints may be used to hasten progress. They include:

1. Serial stretch splints
2. Lively splints
3. Plaster cylinders.

*Serial stretch splinting*

Serial stretch splinting is designed to maintain an

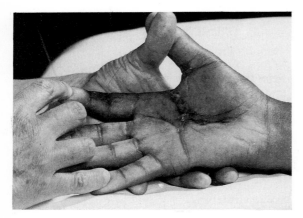

**Fig. 3.15** Support of the MCP joints must be ensured while passively stretching the interphalangeal joints.

equal amount of stretch to that given by the physiotherapist during treatment. The splint should be worn for an hour at a time only. The most suitable time is for a short while following meals, both at midday and in the evening, when the patient is less likely to need the use of both hands. The splint should never stretch more than the physiotherapist has achieved during treatment. The instant the hand or finger is able to lift away from the splint a new one must be made. At the beginning, this change will probably be daily, becoming less frequent as range is increased. Sometimes it is difficult to keep up with the improvement, even with a daily change, but without using this method no improvement is gained at all.

At night a less stretching splint is worn so that any range that has been gained during the day is not lost overnight. The hand is splinted in a comfortable but optimum position which will allow the patient to sleep without being disturbed by pain.

Very thorough and strict instructions should be given to the patient on the use of this technique. Frequently an over-keen patient will use the splint for much too long and cause a painful reaction. Written instructions should be accompanied by a description of the consequences if it is over used.

*Advantages*
1. Patient uses the hand throughout most of the day.
2. Splints are made easily and quickly by the physiotherapist in the department.
3. Tissues are not stretched further than the stretch achieved by the physiotherapist.

*Disadvantages.* The splint must be altered or made afresh rather frequently, possibly daily, but use of thermoplastic materials can make the alterations simple.

*Lively splinting*

Lively splinting is preferred by some physiotherapists as the means to regain loss of finger extension and flexion by using a constant mild elastic or spring stretch.
1. An outrigger is made from Kramer wire or a perforated splinting material such as Hexcelite onto which is looped an elastic band(s) which stretches the stiff finger or joints (p. 116).
2. A Capener splint can similarly be used for

increasing extension of interphalangeal joints (p. 115).
3. Hooks glued to the finger nails can be used to pull the finger tips towards the palm in the direction of the scaphoid using elastic bands. This should help to improve any loss of flexion, particularly in the proximal interphalangeal joints (p. 161).

*Advantages.* These methods will quickly mobilise a joint which has become stiff over a short period of time.

*Disadvantages.* Elastic bands can get in the way of normal hand function, are usually not strong enough to combat persistent joint stiffness and need regular adjustment of tension.

*Plaster cylinders*

Plaster cylinders may succeed when very resistant stiff joints have not responded to any other mobilising technique. The day following application of the cylinder a small piece of cork should be wedged into the plaster to decrease the contracture. This is then worn for a further day or two (p. 114).

Cylinders should not be left on the patient for more than two or three days because of the undesirable effects of immobilising the hand. This method is effective for increasing wrist extension and interphalangeal joint extension when they are unresponsive to other techniques.

*Contraindications to the use of orthoses include:*
1. Articular surface injury.
2. Inflamed joints.

Further details of the manufacture of splints and their materials are given on pp. 102–116.

## Selection of mobilising techniques

The selection of techniques to be used is influenced by various factors such as extent of injury and degree of healing of bones, soft tissues and skin. The diagnosis of intracapsular or extracapsular joint injury is of prime importance.

*Intracapsular injury*

Dislocations and fractures through the articular surfaces of the joint fall into this category. Experience has shown that these joints need careful treatment, and indeed they may never regain a completely full range. Immobilisation should be in the 'safe' position if possible and for the shortest time necessary. Joints are assessed to identify any limited range of active, passive physiological and accessory movements, and also the degree of pain which is produced by any of these movements. Physiotherapy should be introduced gradually in order not to irritate the joint.

The following methods only should be used for treatment of these injuries:

1. Free active movements
2. Accessory movements when the joint is cool and pain-free
3. Gentle functional activities.

All should be monitored carefully. Any increase of pain, decrease of range, or a hot swollen joint will indicate over-treatment. Resistance and strong functional activities should be added gradually when it is seen that there is no reaction to the treatment already commenced

### Extracapsular injury

Most injuries and surgery of the hand will need immobilisation which will tend to produce some temporary joint stiffness even if that joint itself is not damaged. Treatment should commence as soon as the surgeon in charge will allow. Most of the techniques are suitable for treatment but must be selected according to the diagnosis, the findings of the assessment and the time lapse after injury.

## ACTIVE MOVEMENT

All types of active hand function must be restored as quickly as possible after injury. Both the injury itself and any enforced immobility are likely to cause some degree of disability; therefore normal patterns of movement with the correct sensory input should be introduced early for a good recovery. Any delay which is longer than necessary will reduce the chances of regaining total function.

The plasticity of the nervous system is now widely acknowledged, and although the brain mainly recognises patterns of movement it is possible to teach individual muscle contractions, to change the role of muscles, and even to influence the properties of the fast and slow contracting muscle fibres. The density of sensory nerve endings found in the hand offers one of the means by which the physiotherapist should influence the motor response. Stimulation of the proprioceptors enhances the recognition of individual joint movement and the low ratio motor units help in learning to contract muscles individually.

Hand-to-hand contact is a very normal experience in our lives, and it is especially relevant at this stage for the physiotherapist to apply her hands when attempting to improve motor function, thus facilitating all types of exercise. The beneficial effect will not only be physical but also psychological. Patients will find that free active exercises are difficult to perform, especially when the amount of movement is small, as there is very little sensory feedback. If the muscles have been paralysed or immobilised for some time they may have totally lost all knowledge of how to contract efficiently. The maximal sensory input that is safe should therefore be applied. In the early stages only the lightest touch should be used but this can still be extremely effective.

Neuromuscular facilitation concepts (Knott & Voss 1968) should be utilised whether the therapist is working in total patterns of movement or re-educating an individual muscle. Exact positioning and use of the hands are important whatever type of exercise is being given. Traction or approximation of joints, quick stretch to muscles both prior and during contraction, a suitable amount of resistance, irradiation and successive induction are all principles which should be used for re-education and strengthening purposes. Reciprocal relaxation of antagonists and the relaxation which follows maximum contraction of the agonists (Sherrington 1961) are methods which should be utilised where there is adaptive shortening of muscles.

All treatments previously discussed are subordinate to exercising, the most essential part of the treatment programme. Treatment time should be occupied largely by exercises and functional activities in order to regain normal use of the hand. It is easy to get into a habit of using the unaffected side and the patient may need to be prompted frequently so that he quickly regains the automatic response between brain and injured hand.

Complicating factors which may hinder therapeutic exercise are the degree of peripheral nerve (or root) damage, and any other associated involvement such as direct muscle injury, fractures, contractures, adhesions, and skin loss.

## Effects of active exercise

Exercises should be used to reduce oedema, relieve pain, mobilise joints and soft tissue contractures, strengthen or re-educate muscles, re-educate sensation and improve function. One suitable exercise can usually fulfil several of these aims if planned carefully.

### 1. Reduction of oedema

Exercises performed in elevation will help to reduce oedema. Formal exercise sessions with the arm positioned on the raised back-rest of a plinth should follow other treatment methods such as ice, pneumotherapy and pulsed diathermy. Manually resisted exercises to the wrist, hand, fingers and thumb, and the squeezing of foam, Plastazote, balls and grips, are all appropriate. Double Tubigrip finger-stalls or an elasticated glove worn during this elevated exercise will help to accelerate both venous and lymphatic return. The patient should, wherever possible, continue with other elevated activities in the occupational therapy department.

### 2. Relief of pain

Movement is one of the most natural means by which to relieve pain. Frequently, following injury, the pain is caused by increased pressure from oedema, and elevated exercises will help to reduce this (see above). The movement also stimulates the mechanoreceptors and utilises the gate control theory of pain. With the increased activity the sensory input can be gradually returned to normal, so that the pain diminishes and frequently disappears.

### 3. Mobilisation of joints

Active movement, if available, is the best method to maintain and increase joint range. Particular emphasis should be placed on the proximal muscles as the shoulder is liable to stiffen following hand trauma, especially in the elderly.

Stiff joints which are being mobilised with passive physiological movements and passive stretching will improve more rapidly by the addition of active movement. In the author's experience with nerve lesions, a joint which has been difficult to mobilise will frequently regain range at the moment of muscle re-innervation. Conversely, a joint will stiffen more rapidly when immobilised if the muscles which effect the movement of that joint are paralysed. This is especially so when both agonists and antagonists are affected, as the accessory besides the physiological movements are then totally absent.

### 4. Reduction of soft tissue contractures, adaptive shortening of muscles and adherence of scars

Strong muscle action is very effective in stretching the soft tissues which have developed adaptive contractures, e.g. webs. The part should be exercised into the fullest available range and the patient urged to stretch as hard as possible. The muscles may need strengthening in order to utilise their power effectively on any contractures.

Muscle power should also be used for stretching adherent scars which most commonly occur between skin and underlying muscles. A scar on the anterior aspect of wrist and forearm that is bound down onto superficial muscles can prevent both full extension and full active flexion of wrist and fingers. In performing these movements the scar will be seen to shift, being stretched first proximally then distally by the muscles.

The therapist should apply a strong stretch at the moment when the adherence prevents any further range and at the same time command the patient to contract hard. This should be repeated several times.

A second method is for the therapist to place a hand firmly on the skin immediately proximal to the scar and ask the patient to bend wrist and fingers. The scar is stretched when the adherence moves under the strong grasp of the therapist's fingers. In movements into extension the hold should be distal to the adherence. These procedures can be rather uncomfortable for the patient, so that the degree of movement and pressure should be applied gradually.

## 5. Strengthening and re-education of muscles

Muscles which are normal will need maintaining or strengthening and those which have been paralysed or transferred will need re-educating.

a. *Normal muscles.* With a hand injury the proximal muscles quickly weaken without exercise. The musculature of the shoulder and shoulder girdle must be maintained, as the hand cannot function effectively without a stable link between it and the trunk. PNF techniques are particularly suitable for strengthening and helping to retain full diagonal and rotational movements of the shoulder. Active elbow movements together with pronation and supination should be given if the elbow and wrist have not been immobilised in plaster.

The long flexors and extensors of the forearm should be exercised when the muscles are not denervated as a result of a high nerve lesion. Care must be taken when commencing this activity if there has been tendon injury or surgery. Function of the small muscles of the hand will need plenty of attention when the hand itself has been injured. Detailed instruction of individual muscle function should be given to the patient so that he understands how the movement is controlled.

Isometric contractions should be taught within the first few days of immobilisation of fractures and dislocations, or soft tissue injury and surgical repair.

b. *Re-innervated muscles.* When re-innervation is anticipated, following a peripheral nerve lesion, the examination for muscle flickers should be frequent and individual muscle re-education commenced as soon as a flicker is discovered

c. *Re-education of muscles in an altered role.* Following irreversible nerve damage, function can frequently be restored surgically by utilising the tendon of a muscle with normal innervation. This is re-sited into the tendon of the permanently denervated muscle and is termed a tendon transfer. It will need careful re-education to achieve the required change of role (p. 167). Pre-operative treatment is expedient, as it enables the patient to isolate the donor and its action prior to transfer. Complete transposition of muscles together with their neurovascular supply will also need similar re-education.

Occasionally trick movement can be used to provide function when there is permanent nerve damage. This may need re-education, although some patients easily learn the trick by themselves.

## 6. Re-education of sensation

Sensory ability combines most effectively with motor performance, and should always be retrained in a functional manner (p. 98).

## 7. Function

All roles of function should be utilised and retrained if necessary. The habit of using the unaffected side must be corrected quickly and the use of automatic responses and reflexes, games and interesting activities will all help to restore function.

**Methods of exercise**

Activity of each muscle should be assessed and monitored continually, particularly in the presence of a nerve lesion. This is also advisable with other injuries as mechanical defects and unsuspected nerve lesions are quite often identified as the treatment progresses.

To give comprehensive treatment, exercises should proceed through stages that include individual muscle contraction, action of one or more joints, patterns of movement, and functional activities. Each patient will have a personal requirement and not everyone will necessarily require individual muscle re-education.

Movements should be introduced and progressed carefully in the early stages. As a general rule free active exercise may be started within a few days of injury as long as surgical procedures involving nerves and tendons have not been performed. Reciprocal relaxation methods may be utilised within two days after the suture of tendons (Kleinert et al 1973), but active exercising of these tendons should not be undertaken for three to four weeks at least (see Ch. 4). The application of resistance is delayed for another two weeks (total five), and stretching for a further two to three weeks after that (total seven to eight).

The therapist's hand, placed on the moving surface, provides the best means of facilitation. Not only can it alter the degree of pressure from light touch to strong resistance, but it can also alter the direction of that pressure. The planes of movement of fingers and thumb are constantly changing and only the therapist's hand can instantly adapt to all the variations.

All means of physiological facilitation should be utilised for strengthening muscles, both individually and in PNF patterns. Even before any resistance may be applied the light touch of the therapist's hand on a muscle will help to localise the correct muscle contraction.

Treatment given too strenuously in the early stages following injury may possibly prevent healing of damaged tissues, and will probably exacerbate the release of fibrinogen, thus increasing the fibrosis. Little and often is the best motto for regaining hand function, and the patient must be indoctrinated to use his hand continually throughout the day.

## Individual muscle re-education

It has long been realised that man is capable of learning fast and complicated movements of the hand. It is therefore a practical proposition to re-educate muscles individually, as this ensures that every muscle performs its role correctly in the combination of intricate hand movements. The therapist should check that each muscle has normal anatomical action, making sure that if it does become overpowered by stronger muscles when acting in a group situation it is given special individual strengthening. During the recovery stage of a peripheral nerve lesion, when a flicker has been identified, the muscle should be exercised either individually or in as small a group as possible. The most suitable position for exercise is the same as in the testing instructions with the arm resting on a small cantilever table. Activity of each muscle can be checked from these instructions (pp. 30–43).

In the early stages of re-educating the wrist flexors and extensors, gravity should be eliminated by turning the wrist into the mid-position because the weight of the hand can be sufficient to prevent movement from taking place. Finger movements can usually be re-educated in an anti-gravity position because gravitational weight of the fingers is minimal compared to the power of the muscles. Resistance is increased as the power improves. The following facilitating factors should be included for all muscle re-education:

1. Teach the patient the muscle contraction together with the joint-movement on the normal side. Utilise bilateral action.
2. Watch carefully for the same contraction and movement on the affected side and point these out to the patient.
3. Apply quick stretch to the muscle immediately before the attempt at contraction.
4. Apply the hands to the skin surface in the direction of movement, using either light touch or a suitable amount of resistance. This proprioception will give the patient a better 'feel' of what he is attempting.
5. Apply pressure over the muscle itself to facilitate activity. This particularly applies when educating a new role.

The muscles, when very weak and producing only a small amount of movement, will contract best in the outer to middle range. As strength improves so will the excursion, gradually providing movement into the inner range.

## Active joint movement

Muscle activity may have been weakened following injury or immobilisation, although the nerve supply has remained intact. Power can be quickly built up by systematically exercising all joints. The complexity of movement should be increased as ability and strength improve.

### Wrist movements

The patient should first perform single plane wrist movements of flexion, extension and radial and ulnar deviation, with the forearm supported on a table and hand extending beyond the edge. When a diagonal movement is introduced one muscle will perform more strongly than the others.

Extensor carpi ulnaris (ECU) produces a combination of extension and ulnar deviation, which is very important functionally. Abduction of the fingers and thumb when the wrist is held in a neutral position will automatically produce a strong contraction of ECU and abductor pollicis longus in particular. Extensor carpi radialis brevis extends and stabilises the wrist when the fingers are flexed during gripping action.

Exercising with a handle and spring is useful for

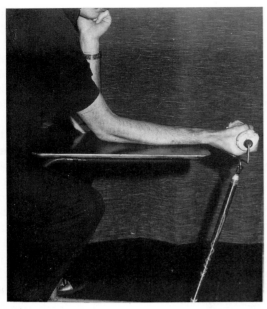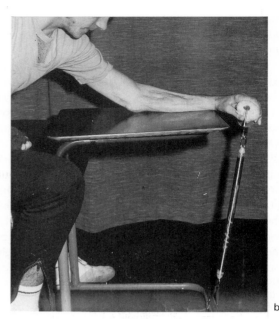

a · b

**Fig. 3.16(a & b)** Patients using a padded handle and spring to improve strength of wrist flexors and extensors. The fingers can be bandaged on to the handle if the flexors are very weak.

strengthening both wrist flexors and extensors (Fig. 3.16 a & b). If a patient has difficulty in maintaining the grasp because the finger flexors are weak, the handle should be padded, and if necessary the fingers bandaged on to the handle. Diagonal movements may be made combining flexion with ulnar deviation, extension with ulnar deviation, and extension with radial deviation. Flexion with radial deviation is a more difficult movement to perform into inner range but is necessary when eating with a fork or spoon or putting food into one's mouth with the fingers.

Frequently after severe hand injury the patients find the combined action of flexing the fingers and extending the wrist quite difficult, and can only flex fingers and wrist together. Use of the handle can be effective in restoring this important pattern of movement.

### Metacarpophalangeal joint movement of the fingers

Flexion, extension, abduction and adduction of the metacarpophalangeal (MCP) joints may be made in isolation or combined with movement of the other finger joints.

*Flexion* of the MCP joints is produced mainly by the interossei which at the same time extend the interphalangeal joints. With palm uppermost the patient should be asked to pull his fingers towards him, flexing at the MCP joints but keeping the rest of the fingers straight (Fig. 3.17). If in the early stages the physiotherapist approximates the MCP

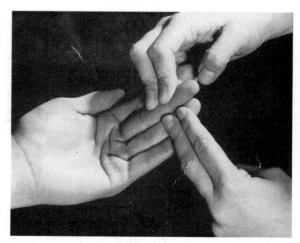

**Fig. 3.17** The fingers being placed in position with some approximation. This facilitates activity of the interossei in the early recovery stage.

joints in this position the muscle action will be facilitated, often enabling the patient to hold the position for a second or so.

Contraction of both flexor digitorum profundus and superficialis will produce secondary flexion at the MCP joints, which is useful functionally when the intrinsic muscles are denervated. This movement is called 'rolling flexion' as it starts at the interphalangeal joints and then 'rolls' into flexion at the MCP joints.

*Extension* movements of the MCP joints should first be taught by keeping the interphalangeal joints flexed and secondly, if possible, by keeping them extended. This latter will depend on the presence of lumbrical muscle activity (see p. 43). Manual resistance should be added as early as possible.

*Abduction and adduction* of the MCP joints are performed most easily with the palm flat on the table or pillow, fingers slightly abducted. The patient is asked to lift one finger, keeping the others in contact with the table, and then to move the finger from side to side. If this is difficult the muscle may be facilitated by applying a quick stretch. The finger is moved by the therapist close to one neighbour, a quick stretch is given and at the same time the patient is asked to move it towards its other neighbour (Fig. 3.18 a & b). A very small amount of resistance is given to the lateral aspect of the moving finger. It will be found that the movement is strongest in its outer range.

As strength improves all the fingers are abducted then adducted together, and resistance can be given by the physiotherapist interlinking her fingers with those of the patient.

### Interphalangeal joint movement

It is usual to exercise both the proximal and distal interphalangeal joints together. There are, however, occasions when it may be necessary to isolate the movement to one joint and to re-educate or strengthen the muscle action of flexor digitorum profundus (FDP) and superficialis (FDS) individually, e.g. tendon sutures or grafts.

*Proximal interphalangeal (PIP) joint flexion* should be re-educated with the palm uppermost on the table. One finger is exercised at a time, and the other three are held on the pillow by the therapist (p. 36). The patient is asked to bend his finger, and the flexion which occurs at the PIP joint only is produced by FDS. This movement may then be resisted. If the distal interphalangeal (DIP) joint flexes at the same time it is likely to be flexor digitorum profundus (FDP) which is producing the movement at the PIP joint and not FDS.

*Distal interphalangeal (DIP) joint flexion* is exercised in the same position, but the middle phalanx of the moving finger is supported firmly by the therapist. The patient is asked to bend the tip of his finger so that FDP flexes the terminal phalanx through range. Resistance is added to the tip of the finger when suitable.

*Combined flexion of MCP, PIP and DIP joints* should be exercised, both with manual resistance

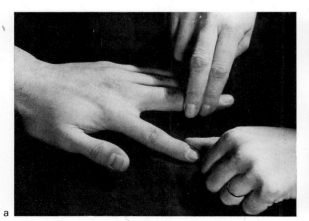
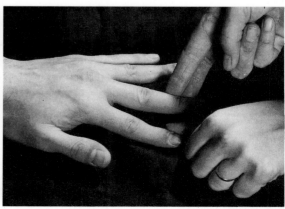

a                                                                                                    b

**Fig. 3.18(a & b)**   The physiotherapist stabilises the index finger, and gives light resistance to the outer range movements of the middle finger.

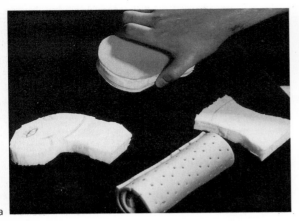
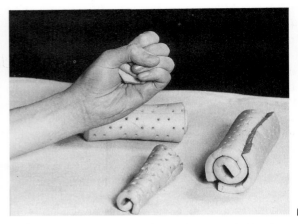

**Fig. 3.19** Varying sizes and shapes of Plastazote for different problems of grasp. (a) Patient had difficulty a week before the photograph was taken in picking up this large piece of Plastazote. (b) The last stage in recovering full finger flexion. Note good PIP joint flexion but limited flexion at MCP joints.

and by grasping objects of suitable size and weight. Differing shapes of foam and Plastazote, such as cylinders and cones, squash and tennis balls, can be given for squeezing. The size and shape must be adapted according to the patient's deformity and power and his ability to produce movement through the whole or limited range. It is very important to get this right as if too small or too large an object is chosen, valuable time and effort may be wasted (Fig. 3.19 a & b).

The combined flexion at these two joints should be strengthened with effort as it is normally a powerful movement. When strong it is particularly useful for regaining range which may have been lost due to injury and immobilisation.

*Interphalangeal joint (IP) extension* is a complex movement and should be re-educated with the metacarpophalangeal joints in both flexion and extension, and also in a combined movement from full finger flexion to full finger extension. This latter can only be produced in a normal pattern when there is activity of both EDC and the lumbricals. Without EDC there is no extension of the MCP joints: without the lumbricals a clawing movement will occur. Extension of the IP joints when combined with flexion of the MCP joints is produced mainly by interossei function (see above).

Due to the changing planes of movement as the fingers extend from fully flexed to fully extended, resistance to both flexion and extension is most

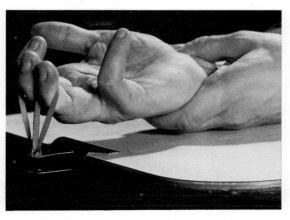
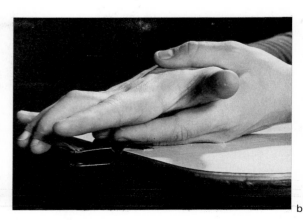

**Fig. 3.20(a & b)** A bull dog-clip with rubber bands attached is useful for strengthening the flexors and extensors of the fingers

easily applied manually. Some resistance using elastic bands looped into a bulldog clip which is fixed to the edge of a table, may be found useful. The patient inserts his fingers into the loops and flexes or extends against the rubber bands (Fig. 3.20 a & b). All activities of grasp and release are beneficial in the early stages of recovery of both extensor digitorum and the intrinsic muscles.

## Thumb movements

Without adequate thumb movement, hand function is extremely limited. A combination of palmar abduction, flexion, opposition and adduction is necessary to achieve an effective grasp of any object. If movement is likely to remain limited the thumb must be positioned in a functional position of palmar abduction and rotation which will allow the finger tips to flex towards it.

*Carpometacarpal (CMC) joint movement*, which is complex as it is a sellar joint, has stability provided by the short but bulky muscles of the thenar eminence.

*Palmar abduction* is necessary in the first place to enable thumb and fingers to part sufficiently to grasp an object. The muscle contraction needs to be fairly powerful to stabilise the thumb and allow flexor pollicis longus (FPL) to flex the distal joints.

Abductor pollicis brevis (APB) abducts the thumb in a plane at right angles to the palm. Its strong activity is extremely valuable in regaining elasticity of the thumb web, which frequently becomes contracted when the muscle is paralysed.

*Opposition* rotates the thumb so that the pulp of the tip, with its special sensory supply, is able to make contact with the object or with the pulp of the index finger. The nail faces away from the tips of the index and middle fingers when the opponens (OPP) is functioning efficiently. It is easier to re-educate this rotational activity in conjunction with the other movements of abduction, flexion and adduction of the thumb.

*Flexion* of the thumb at the CMC by flexor pollicis brevis (FPB) takes the metacarpal across the palm towards the little finger. Without the combined activity with APB this flexion movement would be close against the palm.

*Adduction of the thumb* at the CMC joint by adductor pollicis (Add. P.) provides power for

pinch grip. It also enhances the strength for a normal power grasp.

The therapist can facilitate the activity of these small muscles of the thumb by applying stretch, light touch or resistance with her fingers against the moving side of the thumb.

*Metacarpophalangeal (MCP) joint* movement needs to be as stable as possible in order to perform both light precision movements and strong grasp.

*Flexion* is produced primarily by flexor pollicis brevis (FPB) and secondarily, which is important in a low median nerve lesion, by flexor pollicis longus (FPL). To isolate FPB most easily, the MCP joint is placed in flexion with the IP joint extended and the patient is asked to hold that position. Resistance may be added gradually. FPB is strongly active when the tip of the thumb is opposed to the base of the little finger.

*Extension* is produced by extensor pollicis brevis (EPB) assisted by extensor pollicis longus. Support of the metacarpal enables the patient to localise extension of the MCP joint more easily. Resistance can be given over the proximal phalanx.

*Interphalangeal (IP) joint movement* also needs to be stable as full passive range without active control can be a considerable disability.

*Flexion* is produced by flexor pollicis longus (FPL) and *extension* by extensor pollicis longus (EPL) assisted by abductor pollicis brevis (APB). APB has a slip insertion into the dorsal expansion of the extensor mechanism of the thumb, and therefore in radial nerve lesions when there is paralysis of EPL, it can help to provide some thumb extension.

Both FPL and EPL may be exercised by supporting the proximal phalanx and resisting the movement of the distal phalanx.

*Combination of CMC, MCP and IP joint movements* of the thumb can be produced by asking the patient to make an 'O' with thumb and index finger. When there is little thenar muscle activity a very flat 'D' shape will be produced. As this activity improves the 'D' will broaden and eventually become an 'O'. Activity of the first dorsal interosseous is also necessary during strong pinch grip, in order to stabilise the index finger.

Power should be gradually built up by increasing

the manual resistance. Activities such as picking up objects of different sizes and increasing weight, squeezing foam and Plastazote shapes and balls of different sizes, holding a pole and trying to pull it from an opponent or swinging it from side to side while pronating and supinating the wrist, are all suitable for strengthening grasp.

*Multi-joint movements*

The structures of the hand, with their ability to flatten as a support and to provide arch formations, must be taken into consideration when several joints are exercised together. Extension movements will flatten the arches, while flexion, with opposition of the thumb to the little finger, will assist in the recovery of the arch structures.

Free movements, with their lack of sensory input, are less efficiently performed; therefore manually resisted exercises should be given whenever possible. Nothing can be as effective as the therapist's hands in supplying the resistance at the necessary position and in the desired direction. This is particularly suitable for the fingers with flexion following on into extension and returning once more to flexion (Fig. 3.21 (a & b), Fig. 3.22).

Opposition of the thumb tip towards each of the fingers is facilitated by touch or resistance. A stretch should be given to both thumb and finger away from one another at the start of the movement, and again when the full excursion has been reached in order to increase range and improve power (Fig. 3.23a & b). Ensure that the tip of the index finger also rotates towards the thumb to give an efficient pinch grip. The index has this ability to rotate both towards the thumb and towards the other fingers.

When opposing the little finger tip to the thumb, watch that the 5th metacarpal head is lifting towards the thumb. Without activity of the hypothenar muscles to produce this movement the grasp will be very weak, as found in ulnar nerve lesions.

The patient should be encouraged to use his hands in tapping and striking movements as soon as it is safe (Fig. 3.24). The fingers and hand can be tapped initially onto a pillow, as the impact may otherwise be uncomfortable. Individual finger movements can be performed on the table, first with fingers flat and then flexed, using the tips as in

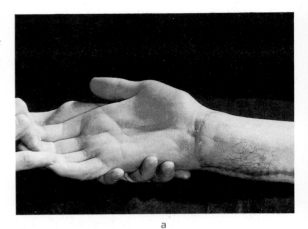

a

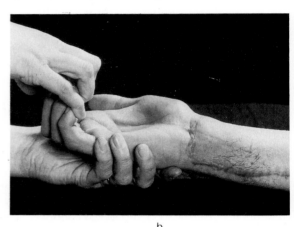

b

**Fig. 3.21** Flexion of the fingers (a) with a quick stretch applied immediately prior to movement and (b) with resistance given.

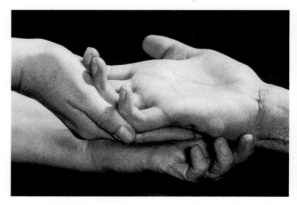

**Fig. 3.22** Extension of the fingers against resistance. Note support given to prevent hyperextension at the MCP joints.

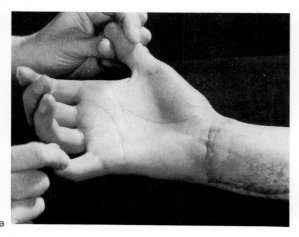
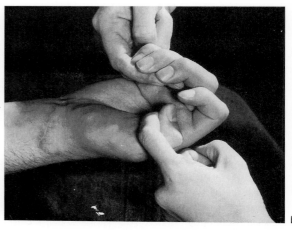

**Fig. 3.23** Attempted opposition of the thumb and little finger towards one another in early stage of recovery after a median and ulnar nerve lesion. (a) Quick stretch applied prior to movement, and (b) light resistance given. Action shown is still mainly from long flexors of thumb and fingers.

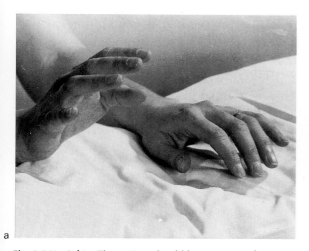
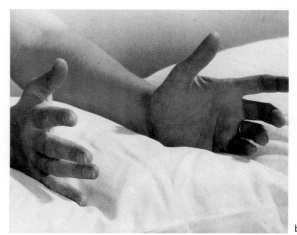

**Fig. 3.24(a & b)** The patient should be encouraged to tap or strike the pillow.

playing the piano. Hand clapping and the tapôtement movements that physiotherapists learn are all suitable when the patient's agility improves and he is less worried by the jarring effect. Games such as pat-a-cake and building up the hands one on top of the other and then placing the bottom hand on top, should be gradually introduced.

Leaning on the hand, either with the whole hand flat or with fingers and thumb tips only, as in positioning a ruler, should be introduced (Figs. 3.25a & b, Fig. 3.26). Pushing movements should be strengthened progressively (Fig. 3.27a

& b). For the elderly it is essential to be able to lean on a hand for support. For young men these movements may be used in press-ups or, more necessarily, to carry out some strenuous work.

There are several advantages to be gained from these activities. Many are bilateral which assists the affected hand in returning to normal, and there is a 'fun' aspect in the competitiveness. For patients who may possibly have a mild algodystrophy or other associated and painful condition they provide a means to stimulate with the maximum normal sensory input, which has probably been

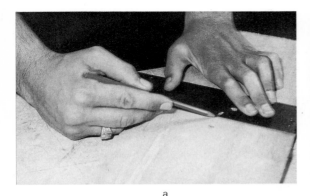

a

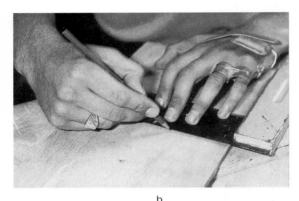

b

**Fig. 3.25(a & b)** Light pressure being.applied to steady the set-square by a patient with a recovering median and ulnar nerve lesion. Note that the splint still corrects a deformity.

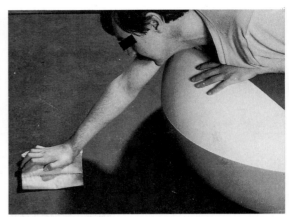

**Fig. 3.26** Weight being transferred on to the heel of the hand. The sand bag conforms to any residual deformity so that the MCP joints are not forced into hyperextension.

missing following injury. Activities must, of course, be modified according to the degree of healing or the pain experienced.

## Proprioceptive neuromuscular facilitation (PNF) techniques

These techniques are an important part of treatment, especially when re-innervation of muscles is occurring after a nerve lesion. They may be performed by the patient using whole arm patterns whilst lying on a plinth, in a modified version

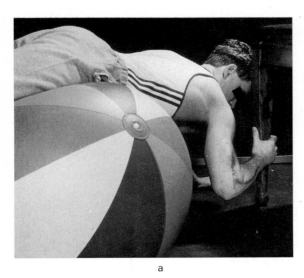

a

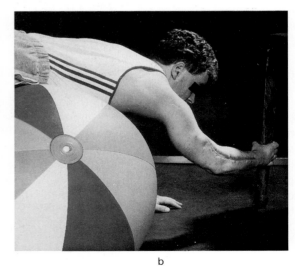

b

**Fig. 3.27** The patient by rolling himself towards and away from the plinth leg is increasing: (a) Extension and (b) Flexion of elbow and wrist joints.

whilst sitting at a table, or when standing.

The patterns of movement used should exploit all the physiological principles which will facilitate muscle activity. These include irradiation of the anterior horn cells, successive induction, use of the stretch reflex, and traction or approximation of joints. Application of the hands on the skin in the direction of movement or over the contracting muscles, giving a suitable resistance, exteroceptive input from the patient's eyes and the therapist's commands, are all ways of achieving maximum sensory input.

Relaxation techniques are useful, particularly when any adaptive shortening of muscles that is due to prolonged immobilisation is treated.

## Lying supine

All patterns may be used, especially for increasing power of the proximal muscles which quite probably are weak from lack of use, and also for strengthening and re-educating the distal muscles of wrist and hand.

## Sitting

During most hand activities we either sit or stand which allows us to see what we are doing. It is very important that the patient is able to watch his movements during re-education of the hand, especially when there is a cutaneous and proprioceptive deficit as a result of a nerve lesion.

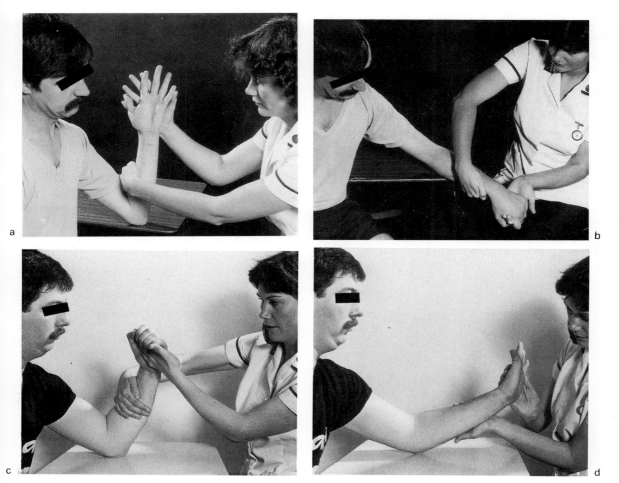

**Fig. 3.28** Modified patterns of PNF pivoting at the elbow joint: (a) Flexion/abduction combines with supination and finger extension (b) Extension/adduction combines with pronation and finger flexion (c) Flexion/adduction combines with supination and finger flexion (d) Extension/abduction combines with pronation and finger extension.

Standard PNF techniques can be modified to be performed in a sitting position. The patient sits at a small table, preferably with an adjustable height; the elbow rests near the edge, either on a pillow or directly on the table top (Figs. 3.28a, b, c & d). The normal patterns of movement are performed in this position with the elbow as the pivot. Little movement can take place at the shoulder joint and full elbow extension is not possible, but the relationship of hand and eye facilitates improved function of the hand.

## Standing

All muscle groups of the upper limb, particularly the shoulder muscles, may be strengthened in the standing and also the sitting position by using the Westminster pulley and handle (Fig. 3.29a & b). The patient's hand should be bandaged on if his grasp is not strong enough for holding the handle.

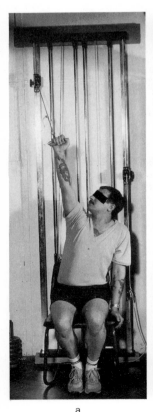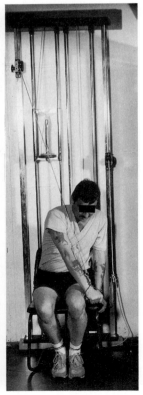

a                    b

**Fig. 3.29(a & b)** The Westminster pulley can be used in either a standing or sitting position.

Padding of orthopaedic felt on the handle will also enable patients with weak finger flexion to hold the handle more firmly. The amount of padding is reduced as soon as flexion improves.

## Main patterns of movement

1. The flexion, abduction and external rotation pattern combines with supination, wrist extension and radial deviation, thumb extension, and extension and abduction of the index and middle fingers in particular. Elbow flexion is incorporated into this pattern when performed in sitting (Fig. 3.28a).
2. The extension, adduction and internal rotation pattern combines with pronation, wrist flexion and ulnar deviation, and flexion of the thumb, index and middle fingers in particular (Fig. 3.28b). Elbow extension is a component of this pattern.
3. The flexion, adduction and external rotation pattern combines with supination, flexion and radial deviation of the wrist, flexion of the thumb, and flexion of the ring and little fingers in particular (Fig. 3.28c). Elbow flexion is incorporated when performed in the sitting position.
4. The extension, abduction and internal rotation pattern combines with pronation, extension and ulnar deviation of the wrist, and extension of the ring and little fingers (Fig. 3.28c). Elbow extension is a part of this pattern.

## Thumb and other finger movements

Variations of thumb and finger movements may be made by slight alteration of the distal components of pattern:

    (i) Extension of the thumb combines with pattern no. 1.

    (ii) Adduction of the thumb combines with pattern no. 3.

    (iii) Opposition of the thumb combines with pattern no. 2.

    (iv) Palmar abduction of the thumb combines with pattern no. 4.

    (v) Extension of IP joints together with flexion of MCP joints of index and middle fingers combines with pattern no. 2 (replacing finger flexion).

(vi) Extension of IP joints with flexion of MCP joints of ring and little fingers combines with pattern no. 3 (replacing finger flexion).

(vii) Abduction of the fingers combines with pattern nos. 1 & 4.

(viii) Adduction of the finger combines with pattern nos. 2 & 3.

## Functional activities

The whole patient and not just the hand itself should be treated from the earliest moment following injury. It is vital that the patient is not allowed to develop the habit of nursing his hand, i.e. never using it, but allowing it to be 'treated' by the physiotherapist. Functional activities, even the easiest of tasks, offer the best means for retaining the normal relationship between brain and hand movements.

In the early stages after hand injury it is recognised that the shoulder, shoulder girdle and elbow should be exercised. These joints should also be exercised bilaterally as this is standard practice in our normal lives. Bilateral patterns of PNF are especially suitable.

Exercising, mobilising the joints and re-educating the muscles are all important adjuncts to treatment, but performing an activity such as picking up a soft ball, squeezing it and putting it down requires a more conscious effort than just squeezing that ball. Problems of non-use should never occur if this approach is commenced early.

Some patients with severe hand injuries find it impossible to perform any activity at all. For example, one young man, with a median and ulnar nerve lesion, was unable to flex his fingers except for a flicker of movement in the nearly fully extended position. By providing him with a suitably-sized piece of Plastazote cut to slightly less width than the distance of his finger to thumb, he was able to pick-up an object for the first time for several weeks. His triumph at his success was enormous, and his morale instantly improved. The size of the Plastazote was reduced daily and his progress became more rapid with the addition of this activity than with exercises alone.

When patients are sufficiently fit following injury, bilateral activities such as bouncing, catching and rolling of large but lightweight balls should be introduced. Beach balls are ideal for this pur-

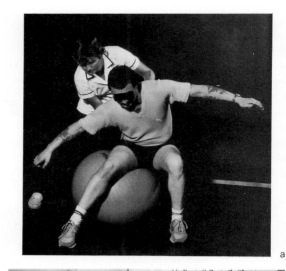

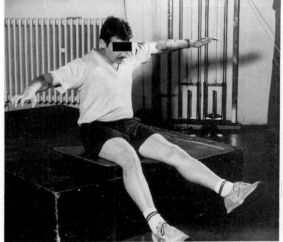

**Fig. 3.30** Balance reactions will assist bilateral re-education when sitting: (a) on a gymnastic ball (b) on a rocker board.

pose. Balance reactions, sitting on a rocker board placed on a low plinth or on a gymnastic ball, should also be practised (Figs. 3.30 a & b). Class work in the gymnasium with other patients who have a variety of upper limb problems forms a most useful part of treatment, both physically and psychologically. Worries and difficulties can be forgotten when a patient joins in games and competitions with others (Fig. 3.31). Specific treatment can be given by careful selection of activities and if necessary the use of adaptations such as padding of handles for table tennis and badminton.

As treatment progresses an increasing number of

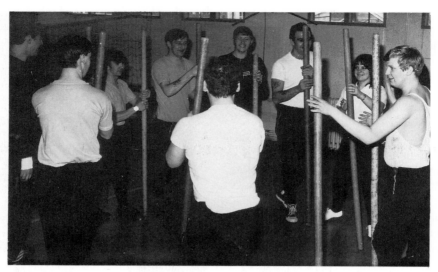

**Fig. 3.31** Worries and difficulties can be forgotten when joining in with others.

suitable activities should be introduced, the selection depending on the patient's problems and his future requirements, his occupation and his leisure interests. Availability of occupational therapy is essential for good rehabilitation and the emphasis should gradually change from formal to functional treatment.

For certain reasons, such as severity of injury, number of operations or even lack of therapy, some patients may not have benefited from this holistic approach. They may already be one-sided, not attempting to make use of the injured hand. Some will 'carry' it in front of them, when they should let it hang and swing naturally by the side. It is imperative that this is quickly corrected. Lack of use should be pointed out to the patient each time it is noticed, with the request to use the affected hand normally.

All the above-mentioned bilateral activities are useful methods of correcting a one-sided habit. However it may be necessary to nag constantly at these patients until they consciously start to use their affected hand. Eventually this use will become automatic.

## Games and activities suitable for use in the physiotherapy department and gym

Some activities are listed which are suitable for the early stages of treatment prior to rehabilitation in the heavy workshop.

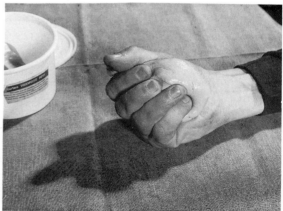

a

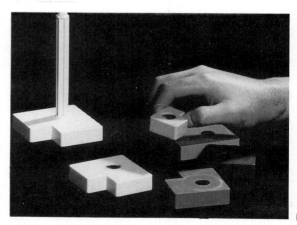

b

**Fig. 3.32** Objects for weak grasp: (a) Silicone putty (b) Children's stacking toys.

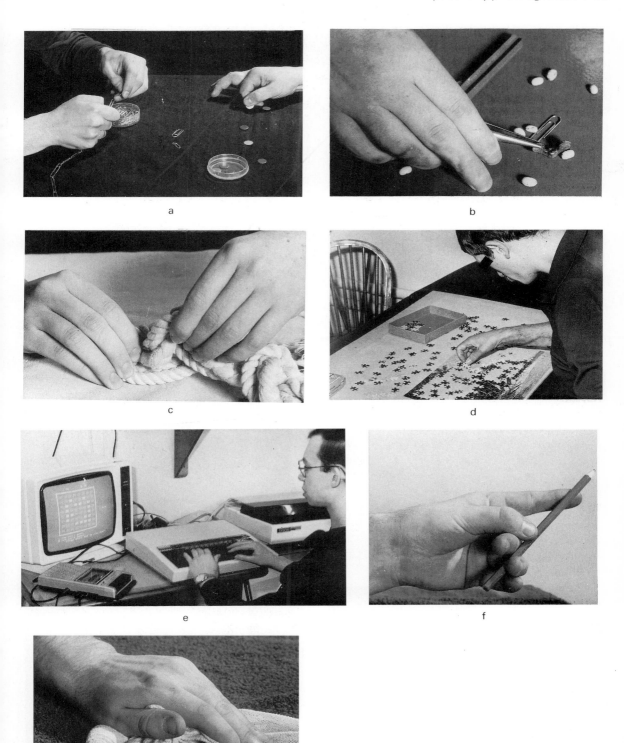

**Fig. 3.33(a–g)** Games and activities for dexterity and intrinsic movements.

## Objects for large but weak grasp

Foam balls
Plastazote cut to shape (Fig. 3.19a)
Plastazote moulded to different shapes and sizes (Fig. 3.19b)
Silicone putty (Fig. 3.32a)
Tennis or squash balls
Cones from cotton yarn
Children's stacking toys, bricks, Tupperware ball, post-box etc. (Fig. 3.32b)
Wooden shapes to fit in board
Large alphabet letters.

## Smaller objects, and games and activities for dexterity

Pik-a-stik
Dominoes, draughts etc.
Tiddly-winks (Fig. 3.33a)
Linking paper clips (Fig. 3.33a)
Pair of forceps to pick up small objects (Fig. 3.33b)

Tying string in knots and untying (Fig. 3.33c)
Jig-saw puzzles (Fig. 3.33d)
Playing cards
Typing or computer games (Fig. 3.33e)
Piano playing
Folding paper and making creases e.g. paper darts
Building matchsticks or plaster of paris reels into towers
Writing, painting
Twiddling a pencil between the fingers (Fig. 3.33f)
Rucking-up a crêpe bandage (Fig. 3.33g).

## Activities for increasing power of flexors

Westminster pulleys
Springs used with handles (Fig. 3.16a)

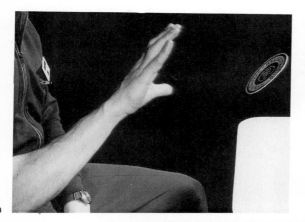

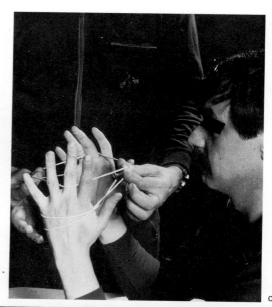

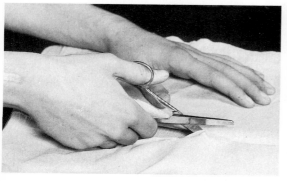

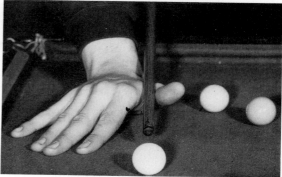

**Fig. 3.34(a–d)** Games and activities for extensor movements.

Rubber bands on bulldog clip (Fig. 3.20a)
Table tennis
Badminton, tennis etc.
Pole games and exercises (weighted or free)
Ball throwing and catching
Multigym.

### Activities for extensors

Springs with handles (Fig. 3.16b)
Jacks
Flipping beer mats (Fig. 3.34a)
Cutting with scissors (Fig. 3.34b)
Cat's cradle (Fig. 3.34c)
Rubber bands on bulldog clips (Fig. 3.20b)
Snooker (Fig. 3.34d)
Yo-Yo.

### Activities for co-ordination

Picking up 5 match sticks (Fig. 3.35)
Pik-a-stik.

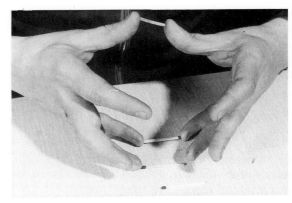

**Fig. 3.35** Activity for co-ordination—picking up five matchsticks.

## Biofeedback

Electromyographic biofeedback, using surface electrodes placed over the motor points, can assist the patient in the early stages of muscle re-innervation when little joint movement or muscle contraction is obvious (Fig. 3.36a). The apparatus can also be linked with a computer which provides a variety of patterns with which the patient may work (Fig. 3.36b). His muscle contraction produces a small visual response, and the stronger the contraction the higher it appears on the screen. By increasing or slightly relaxing the contraction the

**Fig. 3.36** (a) A patient uses EMG bio-feedback with surface electrodes to re-educate his recently reinnervated flexor muscles following a high median and ulnar nerve lesion. (b) The apparatus is linked with a computer programme.

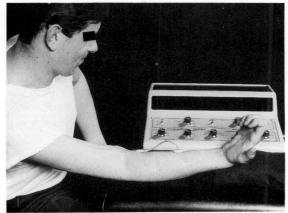

a

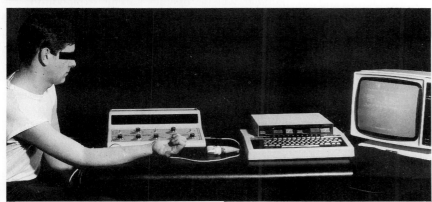

b

patient is able to steer the light response through the patterns, which can be pre-set according to ability. Auditory signals are also available but these may prove aggravating in a busy department. The patient's muscle power can also be recorded for future reference.

## Electrical stimulation

Stimulation is nowadays not used as a standard treatment of muscles paralysed from nerve damage. Insufficient evidence has been provided to substantiate the claim that it prevents muscle fibre wasting. Limb metabolism can be maintained equally effectively if the circulation is good, all available active movement is performed frequently, and the joints, muscles and soft tissues are kept mobile by stretching and manipulating. Stimulation is time consuming and is also very passive treatment, allowing available active movement patterns to fall into disuse. To be effective each muscle would have to be stimulated a hundred times a day, seven days a week without fail.

Electrical stimulation may however be useful in the following circumstances:

1. Immediately following a nerve lesion it is useful in discovering any anomalies of nerve supply to the muscles by stimulating the trunks of the unaffected nerves.
2. Following nerve degeneration and disuse the threshold of the nerve will be raised. A session or two of stimulation can facilitate the muscle contraction because the conduction of electrical stimuli along the nerve has the effect of returning the threshold to a more normal level.
3. Following long-term disuse the idea of movement may be lost. Stimulation combined with the patient's attempt at active contraction may be useful, but should be limited to a few sessions only.
4. After an additional injury, such as falling onto the injured hand, the patient's ability to contract a muscle may be totally inhibited. He may, for instance, be sure that he has ruptured his repaired tendon. Stimulation of the muscle can prove, however, that the tendon is still intact.
5. When EMG facilities are not available it can be useful in differentiating between a neurapraxia

and an axonotmesis by stimulating the nerve trunk distal to the lesion. Two weeks' delay must be given in order to allow the wallerian degeneration to occur in the case of an axonotmesis.
6. Strength duration curves may also be performed to show that muscle re-innervation is occurring. These tests when performed carefully can be very accurate, but are unlikely to show as early results as can be shown by EMG.

## SENSATION

Without adequate sensation the patient is unlikely to use his hand efficiently as there is neither sensory feedback for monitoring the movement nor stereognostic ability. The skill of the brain to interpret sensation correctly is the consequence of proprioception combined with tactile sensation, and this functions most efficiently in a moving situation. Sensation, however, may occasionally be experienced passively, for instance a sting will cause a localised sensation.

## Stages of sensory alteration

With recovery of sensation there is a gradual progression from anaesthesia to hyperaesthesia, followed by either normal sensation or hypoaesthesia. Hyperpathia is an extremely painful response to light touch, but is a fairly uncommon phenomenon.

### Stage of anaesthesia

The presence of total anaesthesia due to nerve damage will necessitate careful explanation: the patient should be warned by the therapist of the inherent dangers. These include burns from a variety of everyday objects such as kettles, saucepans, tea-pots, irons (especially for ulnar nerve anaesthesia) radiators and soup or other hot food. Cold burns may occur from household freezers or carbon dioxide snow, and blisters may eventuate from prolonged friction of anaesthetic skin. Burns will be produced at lower temperatures than usual and, without the normal autonomic response, the blisters and resulting trophic lesions will be slow to heal due to the poor nutrition of the area.

It is not enough to warn the patient once about the dangers of burning his hand. All the possibilities must be spelt out in great detail before he will fully understand the consequences. Regular reminders are therefore essential. He must realise that he has to watch every single movement that he performs, especially when he is near anything hot.

The therapist should advise the patient on the length of time he will probably have to wait before some sensation returns: this will help him cope with what is usually a temporary situation. Most patients will understand the term 'an inch a month' better than 'a millimetre a day', although the latter is a more accurate measure for use by the clinical staff.

### Stage of hyperaesthesia

A pins and needles sensation is the first sign of some sensory regeneration, the hyper-sensitivity being the result of inadequate insulation by the myelin sheaths. As the myelin matures the hyperaesthesia will progressively lessen, but in older people it can frequently remain a problem. Although fine sensory discrimination cannot be achieved at this stage, this hyperaesthesia should provide some sensory protection from heat, cold and friction as it progresses into the hand towards the finger tips.

Test tubes containing hot and cold water can be used to demonstrate temperature recognition, and the patient should be instructed to run his hand slowly over different surfaces, coarse textures and the angles of large objects such as the edge of the table or chair, as an early preliminary to sensory re-education.

The use of TNS as already described (p. 69), may be useful for reducing the unpleasant pins and needles sensation and allow the patient to use his hand more comfortably (Fig. 3.8). Occasionally, however, it has been found to exacerbate the symptoms.

It is now extremely important to encourage the patient to use his hand as normally as possible, for several reasons. Firstly, he must make use of his recovering activity. Secondly, his movement should be 'patterned in' automatically, or he may get out of the habit of using his hand. Thirdly, and most importantly, any sensory in-put from the automatic use will help to modulate any painful afferent discharges.

### Stage of hypoaesthesia and return to normal sensation

As the myelin of the sheaths continues to mature and provide better nerve insulation, so the pins and needles sensation will disappear. It is replaced by sensation which is more normal but which may be reduced, i.e. hypoaesthesia. Not all the sensory neurones will have been able to regenerate to their correct end organs and some may well have regenerated to muscle end-plates. This reduced sensory recovery will produce a 'woolly' feeling. When asked to compare the sensation of the affected limb with the contralateral limb the patient may state that the unaffected side is much more acute than the affected side.

Re-education should be commenced at the stage when the sensation of the palm has returned more or less to normal but the finger tips are still hyperaesthetic.

## Method of sensory re-education

The most appropriate means by which therapists may re-educate sensation is to use stereognosis, or the recognition of objects. This actively involves the patient as he must apply conscious thought whilst manipulating the objects to determine their size, shape, weight, material etc. Not only cutaneous sensation but proprioception will benefit from this method of training and thus improve motor skill.

All tests are performed with the patient's eyes closed or, if necessary, blindfolded. The author prefers not to use the method of putting the hand through an aperture in a screen, as psychologically it separates the patient from his task.

An introductory session to this training is beneficial, in which the therapist asks the patient to describe a large but simple article, continually prompting him by asking about its length and width, the material of which it is made and its weight etc (Fig. 3.37a). This will re-educate him in how to use his various sensory modalities correctly which he may have been unable to do for several weeks, due to anaesthesia. He is then allowed to open his eyes to see whether his description of the object is correct or not.

Articles that are easy to handle should be given

to the patient in the first stage, and those made of different materials will prove easier to recognise, e.g. the bristles and wood of a hairbrush. The objects used for training must not be identical to those used in the assessment. The therapist should not frustrate the patient, either by giving him such small articles that he cannot feel that there is anything in his hand, or by continuing a session for too long. A few minutes several times during the day is found to be most worthwhile.

When the patient has difficulty in recognising an object he should be allowed to handle it in his other

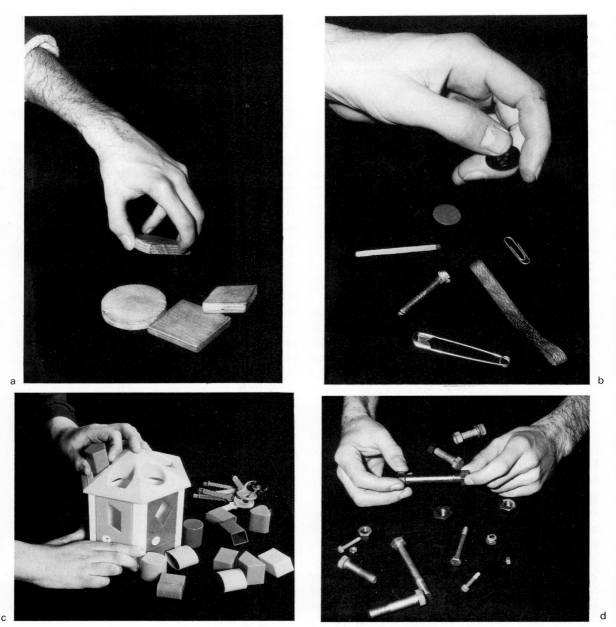

**Fig. 3.37**  Sensory re-education (a) In early stages using different shaped wooden blocks (b) Everyday objects (c) Timed tests of shapes in a post-box. (d) Nuts and bolts.

hand, then open his eyes and look at it. He should manipulate it in his affected hand once more, first while watching and then with his eyes closed. This performance is repeated daily with the same and progressively smaller objects (Fig. 3.37b) and differing types of materials until his repertoire increases and the timing is reduced.

As his sensory awareness improves, the speed and ability of motor performance increases. At this stage it is useful to include tests of speed, with the patient transferring objects from one place, or container, to another, still blindfolded. Timed activities using children's toys, posting shapes into a post-box (Fig. 3.37c), a Tupperware ball with its numerous different-shaped pieces, a board with its cut-out blocks and nuts and bolts (Fig. 3.37d) provide both challenge and interest for patients. Most will rise to the occasion of a contest, particularly if there are several patients undergoing sensory re-education at the same time.

Specific training of proprioception is invaluable, as a considerable degree of gnostic ability is achieved by this means. Patients whose cutaneous supply from the median nerve remains limited can recover reasonable stereognosis and an adequate sensory feedback if their proprioception is particularly efficient. The use of wooden letters (Figs. 3.39 & 3.40) can provide an interesting method in the re-education of this modality.

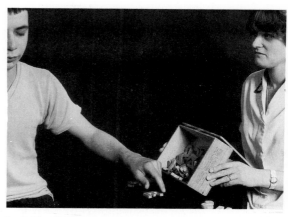

**ig. 3.39**   Finding the correct wooden letters.

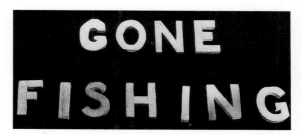

**Fig. 3.40**   A message from the patient to the therapist.

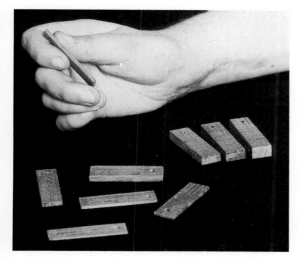

**Fig. 3.38**   Proprioception training with different thicknesses of wood.

## Localisation training

Retraining will usually be necessary after a complete or partial division of a nerve as it is probable that not all the axons will regenerate to their correct end organs following surgery. Localisation may be altered, but training can correct this as long as the patient makes continual functional use of his hand. If localisation is allowed to remain incorrect the patient will receive false information from his finger tips.

The areas of localisation are charted (p. 47) and any incorrect positions are colour ringed. These positions should then be re-educated by the method given below.

A moving finger touch is applied for a couple of seconds over the incorrect area while the patient's eyes are closed. He is then asked to open his eyes and point to the spot where he felt the sensation. If he is correct the therapist proceeds to the next area, but if incorrect the identical spot should again be stroked. This time the patient is asked to open his eyes while the touch is being applied. He watches, and then closes his eyes again for a repeat of the test. He should then be able to say that he knows the spot where he is being touched, but that it still feels like somewhere else. This is the first achievement in the localisation training and it must be continued repetitively over the next few weeks.

Eventually the patient should be able to identify all areas correctly. His improving ability can then be assessed by the speed of identification until an instantaneous correct response is made. The physiotherapist should also 'draw' letters, numbers, shapes and words on the palm and over the palmar surface of the fingers. The patient is asked to name the shape drawn: localisation must be fairly accurate for him to be correct.

Careful initiation into these methods will enable the patient to practise at home. Usually a husband or wife, girlfriend or other suitable person will willingly assist in this treatment when a noticeable improvement usually occurs.

## ORTHOSES

Simple splinting procedures can be of great value in the treatment of hand injuries, rapidly producing results which might otherwise take several weeks to achieve. Furthermore, most splints can be made quickly and easily in a physiotherapy or occupational therapy department, thus avoiding the delays which occur when ordering splints from a prosthetics and orthotics firm.

Before making a splint, thought must be given to the effect it will have on the joints, the structures such as tendons, nerve and blood vessels, and the skin and web spaces. Joints, if splinted for longer than three weeks in the loose-packed position, may stiffen when the capsules and ligaments become irreversibly contracted. Web spaces may be reduced, and other adaptive contractures can result. It is essential to be able to justify both the reason and the position for splinting, as it must never be used unnecessarily.

There are three main purposes for splinting:
1. To provide rest in a good anatomical and physio-

logical position, thus helping to retain mobility of joints when the splint is removed;
2. To stretch contractures and regain joint range
3. To improve function.

For many years the 'position of function' has been considered desirable for both resting splints and immobilisation, but with increased knowledge of the anatomical structure of joints, their physiology and movement, this is largely being replaced by the use of the 'safe position'. Selection is not always a simple matter, and a compromise may be necessary. Joints which are painful due to inflammatory disorders should not be immobilised in the close-packed position, and if adhesions of soft tissues are likely to form post-operatively, the 'position of function' may prove best. The transverse arches which normally flatten only when the metacarpophalangeal joints are extended, must be maintained. Splinting of MCP joints in extension is not advisable other than for short-term stretching of soft tissue contractures.

### Types and uses

The two main types of orthoses are static and dynamic. Attempts have been made to classify splints according to their purpose, such as 'resist' or 'assist', but these terms do not cover all the possible objectives, for example restriction of movement. It is important, however, that an adequate description is given of the aims and type of splint. Examples are given in Figure 3.41.

### Static splints

The uses for these splints include provision of rest, stretch and pressure.

*Resting splints* are commonly utilised to rest and position those joints that are painful because of inflammatory disease. They are useful also for the following purposes:
1. For immobilisation while healing occurs after surgery of tendons and nerves, skin grafting etc.
2. To provide a suitable position that will help to limit contractures as with the burnt hand (Ch. 5).
3. To provide a functional position in the presence of nerve lesions, e.g. a cock-up splint for the

| | Purpose | Type | Means | Material |
|---|---------|------|-------|----------|
| 1 | Relieve pain | Static | Wrist cock-up | Sansplint |
| 2 | Improve thumb function | Dynamic | Pull thumb into palmar abduction | Neoprene |
| 3 | Stretch adherent scarring | Static | Serial extension stretch | Hexcelite |
| 4 | Improve IP extension | Dynamic | Resist MCP extension | Padded tin with wire coils |

**Fig. 3.41** Description of splints.

wrist following a radial nerve lesion. This allows the flexors of the fingers to continue to provide some function.

4. To give protection to any tender or painful spot which is liable to get knocked, e.g. a cuff for the wrist if there is a sensitive neuroma following nerve damage and surgery.
5. To provide immobilisation or support for an unstable or painfully arthrotic joint, allowing mobility of neighbouring joints to be maintained (Fig. 3.42a & b).
6. To rest infected or inflamed soft tissues e.g. tenovaginitis.

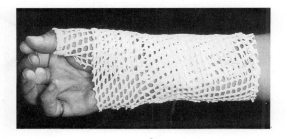

a

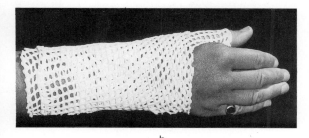

b

**Fig. 3.42(a & b)** Resting splint of Hexcelite for arthritic carpometacarpal joint.

*Stretch splints* can hasten the progress of adaptive shortening, adhesions, contractures and stiff joints. These conditions will usually respond to conservative physiotherapy techniques, but sometimes measurements may show that progress made one day is lost by the next. The principle for the use of these static stretch splints is to maintain the maximum position which the therapist's passive and the patient's own active stretch can achieve. During manufacture the splint must not stretch beyond this achieved position. A splint which maintains this degree of stretch can usually be worn for only 1–1½ hours before it becomes very uncomfortable. Therefore lunch-time, when the patient does not need to use his hand, is found to be the best time as the physiotherapist can apply and remove the splint herself. A check must be made that it is providing the desired effect, that it is not restricting the circulation or producing a localised pressure, and that it is not painful. Careful instruction must be given to the patient prior to its use as frequently an over-keen patient will wear the splint for too long, thus causing a painful reaction.

For night-time use a splint which maintains an optimum position, without giving an actual stretch, will safely ensure that any day-time gains are not lost overnight.

The big advantage of this technique is that the splint is worn for only a short time, allowing the patient to make functional use of his hand for most of the day as it is important that he quickly regains the pattern of normal movement. The stretch of contractures and adhesions may necessitate the hand being positioned in a totally extended or totally flexed position. This would be undesirable for a lengthy period, but is acceptable for very short spells. Mobilisation of stiff joints is the priority, especially in regaining flexion of MCP joints and extension of IP joints. Adaptive shortening of muscles and contracted web spaces also respond well to these splinting techniques, as do superficial adhesions of tendons and skin. Dense adherence of the deeper structures, however, may not be corrected so easily, and prolonged stretching and splinting can cause the joints to become painful. The pain is caused by the big increase of pressure on the joint surfaces that results when strong stretch is applied to the tightly bound-down structures. Surgery is usually necessary to free the tissues when there is no response to intensive treatment.

This type of stretch splinting, as with the passive stretch techniques, should not be used too early as further fibrosis might well ensue. Following tendon and nerve involvement a passive stretch of the damaged structures should not be given until eight weeks after surgery and stretch splinting not for a further two weeks. Splints will need constant changing, sometimes daily, to maintain the same degree of stretch. When kept, numbered and dated they are a visible demonstration of the progress of the patient (Fig. 3.43).

*Pressure orthoses* are particularly effective for superficial problems such as scarring and residual induration of tissues, and also for pain.

1. Hypertrophic scarring following burns and degloving etc. will be reduced considerably by pressure garments, made of Lycra, which must be worn continually for 23 hours a day for a minimum of a year (see p. 185).

Small hypertrophic scars may be treated by the use of a moulded splint of smooth thermoplastic material which is applied to the part with pressure. Make sure, however, that the splint does not interfere with functional movements.

2. Indurated scarring following trauma, particularly when severe, may also be softened by application of pressure from a moulded splint (Fig. 3.44). The pressure decreases any excess fluid in the tissues thus improving movement, reducing fibrosis and ensuring better healing. Polyform is suitable for well-healed areas, and Polymer Resin moulds exactly to deep and tender scars.

Scars in the palm and of both thumb and finger webs are improved by this technique which may also be combined with the application of stretch.

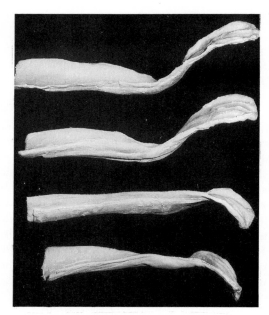

**Fig. 3.43** Serial stretch—visible progress. Note the ridges which hold the fingers in position.

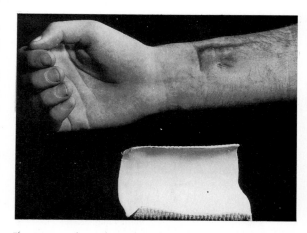

**Fig. 3.44** Indurated scars may be softened by a splint applied with pressure.

3. Bow-stringing of tendons which may have occurred because of a deficiency of the pulley system following tendon injury, suturing or grafting, or damage at the wrist of either the flexor or extensor retinaculum, may be treated conservatively by applying firm pressure to support the tendons in their correct position. The pressure can be provided

by a leather strap round the wrist, or a ring of metal or thermoplastic material round the finger. This method is not always successful, however, as the degree of pressure needed to be effective may possibly restrict the circulation and become very uncomfortable.

4. Pain and tenderness caused by neuromata may sometimes be modified by the application of continuous light pressure using material such as Plastazote which has been moulded on the part (see p. 129). It is held in position by a strap or with Tubigrip. The gate control theory probably explains the reduction of pain with the low threshold mechanoreceptors being stimulated by the pressure. Protection from knocks is also provided over the tender areas.

*Dynamic splints*

These can be used for a variety of purposes including prevention and correction of deformities and replacement and improvement of function. Whenever possible they should be custom-made for the patient.

1. *To prevent deformities.* During the paralysis stage of peripheral nerve lesions, when the normal tone of one muscle group is opposed by muscles that are paralysed, a deformity is likely to develop. Lively splints can prevent this deformity from becoming excessive and at the same time improve function. For instance in combined median and ulnar lesions a wire 'knuckleduster' type splint can prevent hyperextension of the MCP joints and at the same time enable active interphalangeal joint extension to take place.

2. *To replace function.* The power of a dynamic splint can be used to replace the activity of a paralysed muscle. The antagonist must be strong enough to contract against that power. This principle is used in lively splintage for most nerve lesions. For example in a radial nerve lesion a spider splint can provide finger extension.

Positioning with the use of the lively splintage can also enable alternative muscles to provide function. For example in a median nerve lesion at the level of the wrist, the thumb can be pulled into palmar abduction and opposition by a strip of neoprene. Contact can then be made between the tips of the thumb and index and middle fingers by contracting flexor pollicis longus (see p. 148).

Dynamic splinting can also be used to replace activity of a muscle which needs to be immobilised or rested. Kleinert et al (1973) devised the means to rest the long flexor tendons of the fingers following division and primary suture. A rubber band, fixed between the flexor aspect of the wrist and a hook glued onto the finger nail, will hold the finger in a flexed position. The patient can extend his finger against the band, which produces a reflex reciprocal relaxation of the damaged flexor. This daily movement, commenced early after operation, is designed to prevent adhesions forming between the tendon and sheath (see p. 161). It must, however, be very carefully managed for the duration of its use.

The movement of the neighbour finger can be utilised by linking it with the affected digit. This is useful when movement patterns become lost and the patient does not use his finger because muscles are paralysed and the finger sticks out and gets in the way; it is also useful in the early stages following injury when the neighbour can help protect the affected finger. Double Tubigrip may be sufficiently strong and is easily removed and replaced, whereas strapping at the mid-shaft level of the phalanges is stronger but more permanent. A double finger-stall of leather may be used but has the disadvantage of covering the skin so that sensory input is severely reduced (Fig. 3.45a & b).

3. *To strengthen movement.* Application of a mild resistance may be used to strengthen movements that are slow to increase power. Elastic bands suspended from an outrigger or a spring wire splint can give resistance during treatment, but the position of the splint should not be allowed to limit function for long.

4. *To stabilise and restrict movement.* A variety of injuries may occur in the hand which will require some immobilisation. At the same time the urgent need is to keep the rest of the hand and its joints as mobile as possible. Some joint injuries need a stopping devise to prevent full range from occurring and yet encourage a certain degree of movement, as in volar plate injuries (Fig. 3.46). The neighbour finger can be used to give extra stability by strapping the two digits together with elastoplast.

5. *To correct deformities.* Varying degrees of force may be used to stretch deformities. An elastic

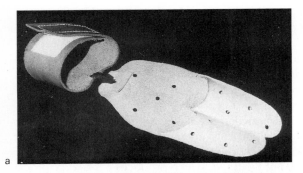

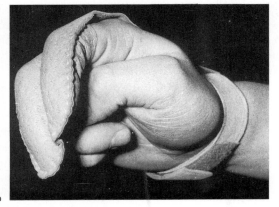

**Fig. 3.45(a & b)**  A double finger stall can assist in the flexion of a finger which might otherwise get in the way.

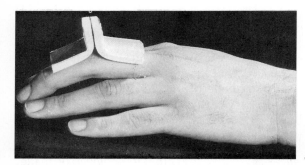

**Fig. 3.46**  A splinting device to restrict full extension following volar plate injury.

band will give a very mild amount of stretch when it is considered safe to apply tension to damaged structures. This can be suspended from an outrigger and attached by leather loops around the finger. Extra elastic bands can be attached later to give increased stretch. The finger can actively flex against the band, allowing functional movement. It is an effective method if used early after lacerations and joint involvement when immobilisation may have produced mild contractures, and it is particularly useful if the extensors are paralysed and unable to correct the deformity actively.

Spring wire splints can be used to correct the more persistent deformities. The strength of the splint can be controlled by varying the thickness of the wire and the number of coils which form the hinges. A Capener splint (Capener 1967) is especially useful for correcting a flexion deformity in the proximal interphalangeal joint of the finger. It can be purchased ready-made in various sizes if not easily constructed in the OT department or workshops.

The power of the dynamic stretch is more difficult to assess, and very great care must therefore be taken that no adverse reaction occurs in the joints or tissues from this type of splinting. Regular monitoring of the hand is essential while the splint is worn.

### Equipment

For the physiotherapist's purposes equipment can be simple (Fig. 3.47) and should include:

   (i)  A plastazote oven (found in most departments)
  (ii)  A pan for hot water (preferably thermostatic)
 (iii)  Bucket and bowls
 (iv)  Scissors and knife
  (v)  Tubigauze and crepe bandage
 (vi)  Paper and chinagraph pencil
(vii)  Vaseline

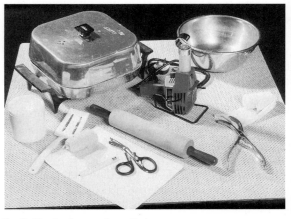

**Fig. 3.47**  Equipment for splinting.

(viii)  Paper towels
 (ix)  Fish slice and rolling pin
  (x)  Heat-gun (not essential).

### Accessories

 (i)  Lining materials
(ii)  Straps and buckles.

### Materials

A wide variety of splinting materials is on the market and the choice will depend on certain needs and requirements. The following give a coverage for most purposes.

#### Plaster of Paris

This is still a practical and general purpose material which is available in most departments. It is cheap, and is made quickly, with the wet plaster moulding intimately to skin creases and the crevices between the fingers without the need of a lining. It is easy to use as the cotton in the plaster does not stretch. It will not, however, mould round contours such as the thumb web unless built up by the application, one after another, of small squares of the plaster.

It is a particularly efficient material for serial stretch splinting as the wet plaster can be ridged between the fingers, thus holding the desired position exactly. Ridges of extra plaster easily added longitudinally to the exterior of the splint, will reinforce it if required for a particularly strong stretch.

The disadvantages include the length of time that the material takes to dry (6 hours or more). It should not be used for a strong stretch whilst damp as it will probably crack. The splint cannot be altered once made, it must be bandaged in position as it is difficult to attach any fastenings and it must not be immersed in water.

#### Thermoplastic materials

These materials are heated by immersing in hot water, preferably in a thermostatically controlled pan, and are applied directly on to the skin of the patient for moulding (Swan 1984). Once a splint has been made it can usually be altered by reheating and remoulding to the desired position.

Most materials can be self-reinforced and straps of nylon and Velcro easily attached by welding them with small pieces of the same material to the splints. The surface may need roughening with sand-paper for the weld to be adherent.

*Sansplint and Orthoplast* are useful materials for making resting splints which do not need to conform round extreme contours. They are fairly rigid once made and are washable.

*Sansplint XR* is more stretchable than plain Sansplint and conforms to most contours. It has a rubber content which prevents overstretching and is therefore an easy material to handle when making the larger gutter-type splints for forearm and hand. It will need reinforcement if used for strong stretch but it can be remoulded and is washable.

*Polyform* is the most stretchable of the thermoplastic materials, becoming soft like plasticine when heated. It can be squeezed into a ball and rolled out like pastry so that all the unused corners of the original sheet can be utilised and the material of discarded splints used again.

Because of this soft consistency when warm it totally conforms to parts such as thumb and finger webs and into any deep scarring. It is a rigid material when cold and is washable. It can be moulded again but is inclined to stretch, become thin and lose its shape at the second moulding. In large pieces it is difficult to manage and the therapist's fingers can easily poke through the material. Its most advantageous use, therefore, is for small splints.

*Aquaplast* has been used extensively for splinting of burns in the early stages to prevent contractures and hypertrophic scarring. It becomes translucent at the correct temperature for moulding, and conforms around extensive contours. It has a memory when reheated so that it returns to its original cut-out shape, allowing a further moulding to be made. It shrinks slightly as it cools.

*Hexcelite* is a versatile material that is supplied both in sheet and strip form. It is a loose cotton mesh, coated with thermoplastic material, and therefore has excellent comformability. It does not overstretch and can be returned to its original shape on reheating except for the folds of the material which have already been welded together by heating and the application of pressure. It can be made into a cylinder and safely immersed in water.

The mesh is useful for attachments and is cool

for summer use. It needs a lining when used over bony pressure points, but can be used unlined for other areas. The initial preparation takes longer as the edges are sharp when cut and therefore need to be turned in and welded by applying pressure with a rolling pin. Once made it can be remoulded any number of times. Reinforcement by the welding of an extra layer or two will produce an extremely strong splint. Straps can also be attached by welding.

*Plastozote* is an expanded polystyrene material that can be used for cylinder wrist supports and for providing a lining for a splint when either the circulation or the skin viability is poor. It is particularly suitable for improving the web spaces in the early stages following severe burns to the hand. The foam material ensures that vulnerable areas will not be pressurized.

Plastazote can be reinforced by strips of Vitrathene welded to it. An oven is a necessity for heating purposes, but with care the Plastazote can be moulded directly onto the patient.

### Serial stretch splinting

The aims of this splinting technique are firstly to improve joint range and secondly to stretch soft tissue contractures, adherence and web spaces. When passive joint range is limited the priorities are to regain metacarpophalangeal joint flexion followed by extension of wrist and interphalangeal joints. These are the movements which are most vital for function and most difficult to recover. They must therefore be tackled first. Splints can also help to prevent the occurrence of contractures, if this seems to be happening, by using them without application of stretch.

It is advisable that passive stretching be carried out for at least a week prior to commencement of splinting so that the physiotherapist knows how much stretch can be safely applied. Post-operative healing of structures such as tendon and nerves must be assured, and it is essential that extension is never regained at the expense of flexion.

Examples of preparation, moulding and application of some of the more frequently used stretch splints are given.

### Preparation

The patient should have his regular treatment of

stretching and exercising immediately prior to splint making, and the same therapist should make the splint. Regular measurements must be taken in order to evaluate the results.

Patterns of a variety of splints can be found in manufacturers' manuals and in textbooks on splinting, which should help the therapist to produce the desired result (Malick 1979).

An outline of the splint can be drawn by placing the hand on a sheet of paper over a pillow or sand bag. The latter can be plumped up into a shape suitable to support most deformities. A paper towel which stretches slightly may be preferred for the pattern, and plasticine can be used as a template when a particularly complicated shape with awkward contours is to be splinted. Unless a paddle splint is being made a crescent should be drawn round the thenar emminence to prevent the thumb being flattened by the splint.

The shape is then transcribed onto the selected thermoplastic material and cut out, allowing a little extra which may be trimmed later. It can be reinforced afterwards by adding another layer or a strip of extra material. Plaster of Paris, if used, requires 12 to 14 thicknesses, reinforced immediately it has set by adding lengthwise ridges of plaster to make a durable strength splint. It is preferable not to use a lining if a really conforming splint is required. Hairy skin should be lightly greased with petroleum jelly to prevent any painful adherence to plaster of Paris. Bony points and tender pressure areas should have a small piece of adhesive felt placed on the skin. This will form a hollow in the splint and the hollow may be either left as it is or padded with a soft material thus preventing painful pressure or friction.

### Moulding

The help of a second physiotherapist is very often needed initially to help position all the joints correctly. A crêpe bandage and the patient's other hand are useful for keeping the material in position on the forearm while it sets or hardens.

### 1. To regain extension

Contracture and adherence of structures on the flexor aspect, which respond well to splinting, are relatively common with hand injuries. A stretch splint is therefore quite frequently required and is reasonably simple to make.

The patient sits with hand supported on a pillow, palm uppermost, and the degree of stretch and position required is checked by the therapist. The splint should extend from the mid-forearm, to give adequate wrist support, and protrude slightly beyond the finger-tips. The width at finger level must be generous enough to ensure that the fingers are not squeezed together. A crescent is cut out for the thenar eminence.

If plaster of Paris is used, the prepared layers are held by the therapist at either end and folded in on themselves. The material is then dipped into a bucket or bowl of water which should be tepid to hasten the setting time. When fully saturated it is squeezed out and unfolded, and there is sufficient time to smooth out any wrinkles before placing the plaster on the patient. It is then moulded to the desired shape of the hand, with some ridges pressed in between the fingers to prevent any slide when the splint is used. Stretch is then applied until the plaster sets. Thermoplastic materials are removed from the pan of hot water, patted dry and similarly smoothed into position and the stretch applied until cool.

The therapist should ensure that the middle finger is in correct alignment with both the metacarpal and the mid-line of the forearm. The transverse arches should be maintained by the splint, unless the hand is fully extended, and the thumb allowed to rest in the functional position.

Just before the material sets the hand should be turned over and the stretch applied in the pronated position; otherwise, when he wears the splint, the patient can relax the tension by pronating his hand (Fig. 3.48a). The hardening of thermoplastic material may be hastened by wrapping a cold wet towel round the splint; immediately it is removed it should be dipped into iced water.

If full extension of both wrist and fingers at the same time is not possible because of adherence of structures, a decision must be made whether to extend the wrist fully and let the fingers flex, or extend the fingers and allow the wrist to flex. Either method should be equally effective if all the joints are fully mobile passively. If, however, the passive extension of one joint is not full it is this joint which should be extended by the splint. Alternating the stretch will be of greatest value when many joints are limited in their passive range. The wrist and interphalangeal joints are those most likely to need attention for regaining extension. Splints must be altered or renewed immediately they become slack. A series will show any improvement made (Fig. 3.48b).

Care must be taken not to hyperextend the metacarpophalangeal joints, especially with an ulnar or a combined median and ulnar nerve lesion.

### 2. To regain web spaces

The thumb web, especially, may need stretching following a hand injury. Plastazote is suitable for very restricted web spaces and those which are painful on pressure and have a poor circulation (Fig. 3.49a). Small wedges or several thin layers

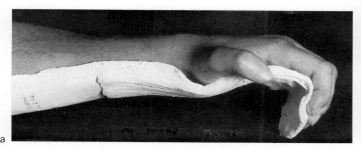
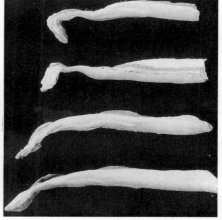

**Fig. 3.48** (a) A stretch splint used for a severe Volkmann's contracture, which is affecting the flexors and also the thumb extensors. Note the poor position of the thumb. (b) The series showing progression towards wrist and finger extension.

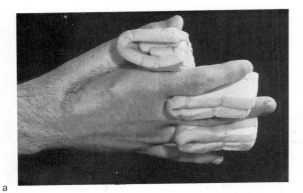

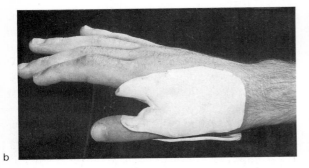

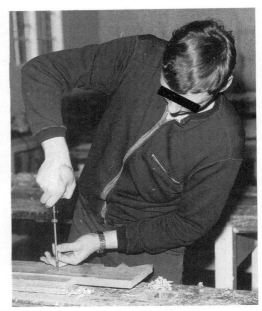

**Fig. 3.49** Tight webs following an explosive injury with a deep scar in the thumb web. (a) Early stretching with Plastazote. (b) Use of Polyform. (c) Patient back to work as a carpenter following the release of scarring and skin grafting.

may be moulded into the web spaces, taking care that the heated Plastazote does not burn the skin.

Polyform is the ultimate choice of material for splinting the thumb web because it will hold the thumb in the desired position better than Plastazote. It conforms exactly to the web shape, but skin and circulation must be sound before a decision is made to use it (Fig. 3.49a, b & c).

A strip of Polyform, 12 cm by 8 cm approximately for an adult hand, is laid in the web; the stretch is gently increased and held steady until the material cools. Care must be taken that the stretch is firmly into the web and does not put a lateral strain on the MCP joints of thumb and index finger.

Palmar abduction with rotation is usually the most essential position to regain, followed by radial abduction. When the thumb web is tight there is a tendency for the thumb to spring back into extension, and if this is so Polyform is the best material to hold the desired position (Fig. 3.49b).

### 3. To regain flexion of the metacarpophalangeal joints

The metacarpophalangeal joints are prone to stiffen in extension, particularly after severe oedema of the hand. They will probably be difficult to mobilise, but serial splinting techniques can usually hasten progress.

Two stages may be required, firstly to regain 60° of MCP joint flexion and secondly to increase from 60° to full flexion. Experience has proved that using a dorsal slab is not only ineffective but it is also very uncomfortable to wear. The volar slab method is more comfortable and can succeed in improving range.

*Stage one* involves making a mid-forearm to finger tip length volar slab. The splint is made with the patient's forearm supinated, palm uppermost and the MCP joints stretched into the maximum flexion.

*Stage two* after 60° has been achieved, incorporates a splint in two parts: i.e., firstly, a wrist cock-up with protruding metal bar at wrist level, and secondly a dorsal pad over which pressure is applied (Fig. 3.50a and b). A crêpe bandage is used to pull the fingers into flexion by winding it first over the dorsal pad and then around the metal post. An effective stretch of the MCP joints can thus be made (Fig. 3.50c) with the fingers flexed also if desired (Fig. 3.50d).

A 2 cm wide and 8 cm long piece of metal (thick

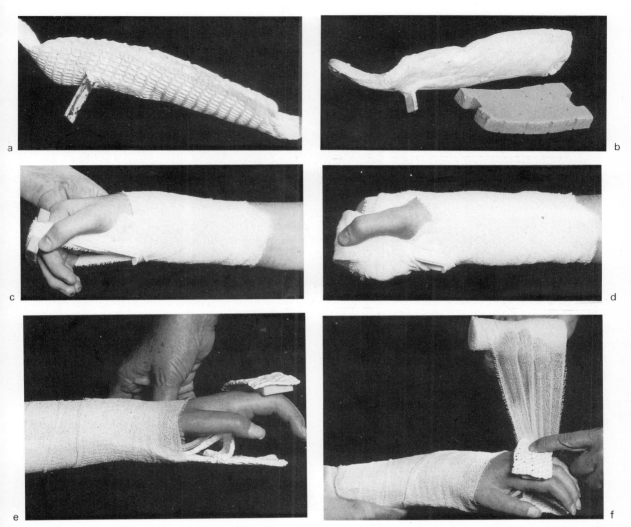

**Fig. 3.50** To regain flexion of the metacarpophalangeal joints. (a) & (b) A cock-up splint of Hexcelite or plaster of Paris with metal post is used together with a slab of reinforced Plastazote. (c) The proximal phalanges are bandaged down towards the metal post and (d) the fingers can be totally flexed with the bandage if desired. (e) An extended cock-up is made when the MCP joints are exceptionally stiff, as in this plexus lesion. (f) The fingers are then bandaged down towards the extension piece.

aluminium or steel) is bent to an 'L' shape of 3.5 cm and 4.5 cm respectively. Most workshops can supply this bar. If plaster of Paris is used for the cock-up splint, approximately six layers of plaster should be applied first.

The wrist should be positioned in a few degrees of extension. Care must be taken that the splint does not extend distally further than the proximal palmar crease (the mid-shaft of the metacarpals), as it would otherwise prevent flexion of the MCP joint (Fig. 3.51). The L shaped bar, short end pro-

truding, is then positioned on the outside of the plaster at wrist level. A slit or a hole is made into the middle of the remaining layers, again at wrist level, before these are moulded over the outside to hold the bar in position. If thermoplastic material is being used an extra piece of the same material should be used to weld the bar to the outside of the splint.

Plastazote may be moulded on the patient for the dorsal pad, but it will need some reinforcement of Vitrathene. Contourfoam, which moulds easily and exactly, is a particularly suitable material for

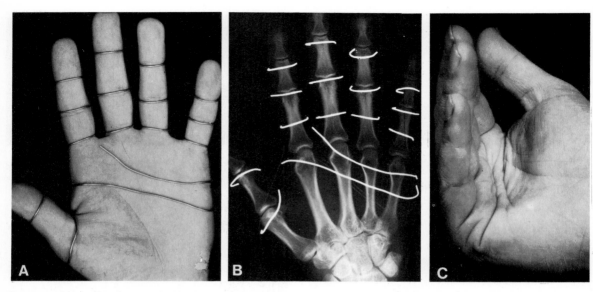

**Fig. 3.51(a, b & c)** Outlines of the hand. The cock-up splint must never extend beyond the proximal palmar crease (mid-shaft of the metacarpals) as it would otherwise prevent flexion of the MCP joints (from Lister 1984 The hand, 2nd edn. Churchill Livingstone).

this purpose and needs no reinforcement. The pad must be wide and deep enough to span the dorsum of the fingers, without squeezing them together, and thus provide a comfortable surface over which the tension of the bandage may be applied.

### 4. To stretch an intrinsic contracture

A cock-up splint should be made which extends as far as the mid-shaft level of the proximal phalanges. This *must* be exact for each finger. The distal end of the splint should be thickened by doubling over

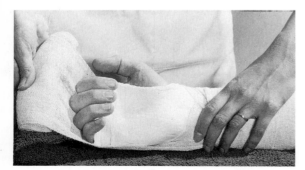

**Fig. 3.52** An intrinsic contracture should be splinted into this position if possible, with MCP joints extended and IP joints flexed.

the last half inch of material while it is still soft. The splint must maintain the metacarpophalangeal joints in extension if at all possible (Fig. 3.52).

When applying the splint the fingers are flexed at the interphalangeal joints over the end of the splint and the bandage is applied firmly round the outside of the finger. Extra padding may be found necessary on the volar surface of the fingers.

### Application of splints

The wearing of these splints must be limited to short sessions only which allows the patient to make maximum functional use of his hand. The most recently made stretch splint, if applied immediately after lunch and after tea, can usually be worn without undue discomfort for one hour. This enables the therapist to examine the hand when the splint is removed after lunch to check the pressure points.

An extremely thin layer of cotton wool should be placed over the splint, which makes it comfortable for the patient to wear and yet allows the ridges and contours to hold the position effectively. A crêpe bandage, wound first round the wrist and forearm, fixes the splint and allows the therapist to position the fingers correctly. These are then bandaged firmly and comfortably onto the splint with the tips exposed to enable a check of the circulation. The fingers should be spread slightly apart and not allowed to drift together laterally. A small piece of cotton wool placed between each finger may help to achieve this spread. The tips of the fingers should never protrude over the end of the splint.

The previously-made splint is usually suitable for wear at night. By maintaining an optimum position only and not giving an uncomfortable stretch, the patient should not be kept awake at night by pain. This maintenance should be sufficient to prevent the occurrence of any contracture of tissues which can easily return the limb to its previous day's position.

Experience has shown that it is preferable to start these stretch splint techniques with the patient living in for a few days. The correct routine is instituted and the patient can then continue to use the splints safely at home. Out-patients who tend to think that the longer they wear the splint the faster they will recover, often exceed the recommended splinting time and return the next day with a painful, over-stretched hand.

Careful instructions must be given to the patient about applying the splint and checking the circulation of the finger tips by colour and temperature. The splint must be taken off if painful, and another less stretching one made, but some discomfort for a short while is found bearable by most patients. Written instructions should always be supplied to out-patients, giving times and length of wear, the precautions to be taken and the care of the splint. This reinforcement by written instruction is usually heeded where verbal ones are either forgotten or disregarded.

## Plaster cylinders

Some joints are particularly resistant to the recovery of full extension, e.g. wrist and interphalangeal joints, but may respond to the use of plaster cylinders (Fig. 3.53a). The cylinder should not be left on the patient for more than 2–3 days without removal for mobilising.

The strength of a finger cylinder must be in the narrow slabs (approximately 3 thicknesses of plaster) which are applied on both palmar and volar surfaces (Fig. 3.53b). Only a small amount of plaster is wound round the finger as this allows the cylinder

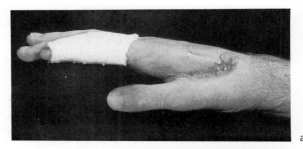

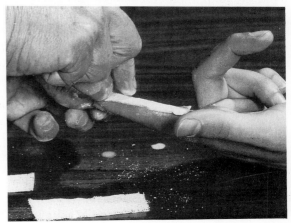

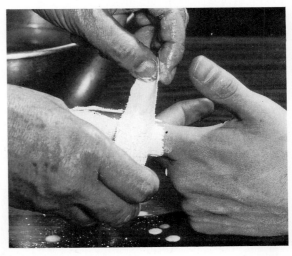

**Fig. 3.53**  (a) A plaster cylinder for regaining full extension of the proximal interphalangeal joint. (b) The cylinder being made with volar and dorsal slabs. (c) A small amount of plaster is bandaged around the finger.

to be cut off easily (Fig. 3.53c). The cylinder should be removed the following day, the finger treated and exercised, and another applied.

Alternatively, once the plaster is dry the cylinder may be wedged without removing it. A cut, the full depth of the plaster, should be made carefully across the volar surface at the level of the flexed joint. Both finger and cylinder are then stretched into some more extension and a small piece of cork squeezed into the gap that appears. A little more plaster is applied over the outside, thus maintaining the extra extension. The next day the cylinder should be removed and the process started again.

A similar method may be used for the wrist joint. Experience has shown that extension, which is usually of greater functional value than flexion, is more difficult to regain. The use of these cylinders has proved to be an effective means to increase range.

### Dynamic or lively splinting

Lively splints may fulfil requirements that cannot be provided by static means. They should be made individually by preference (Fig. 3.54) but a selection of ready-made splints is now available on the market. If used these must be checked carefully for their fit and for their effect on both the anatomy of the hand and its function. Some splints flatten the arches, flatten the thumb, hyperextend the metacarpophalangeal joints and, because they are cumbersome, hinder function.

A few examples of lively splints follow.

1. The position of the thumb in a median nerve lesion can be improved by a Neoprene strip (Fig. 3.55a and b).

A strip approximately 2 cm by 38 cm has a loop stitched at one end. The loop must fit firmly down over the metacarpophalangeal joint. Some of the width may need to be trimmed if it is uncomfortable over the thumb web. The thumb is then pulled into some palmar abduction with rotation, the strip wound round the wrist and fastened on itself with Velcro. The pull on the thumb must come from the ulnar side of the wrist immediately proximal to the pisiform. The thumb is thereby positioned so that

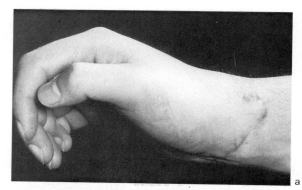

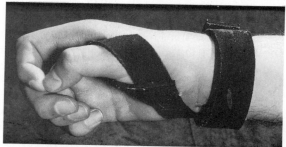

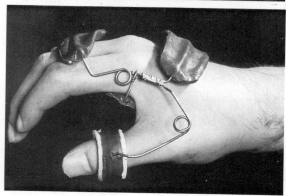

**Fig. 3.55** (a) The position of a tightly adducted thumb following a median and ulnar nerve lesion (b) can be improved by a strip of Neoprene looped and pulled down firmly over the metacarpophalangeal joint. (c) The same patient wearing a coiled wire splint which prevents hyperextension of the metacarpophalangeal joints and positions his thumb effectively.

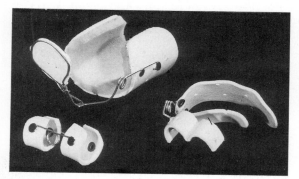

**Fig. 3.54** A selection of lively splints made with the spring wire rivetted to thermoplastic material.

when flexor pollicis longus contracts, contact is made by it with the tips of the flexed index and middle fingers. EPL can extend the thumb against the Neoprene, but when all muscles are relaxed it will be returned to the abducted position.

2. Prevention of hyperextension of metacarpophalangeal joints of the fingers in ulnar and combined ulnar and median nerve lesions: this is most effective when using wire coil splints (Fig. 3.55c). Ideally they should be custom-made, and details of their manufacture are given by Wynn Parry (1981).

The positioning of the MCP joints in slight flexion enables extensor digitorum to extend the IP joints. In the combined median and ulnar splint a wire extension piece places the thumb in the functional position of palmar abduction (Fig. 3.55c).

3. Active finger and thumb extension, if absent due to radial nerve damage, can be replaced efficiently by a spider splint. One end of this commercially-produced splint, which comes in three sizes for each hand, loops over the thumb. Four spring wires, with a cup at the end of each, radiate in a curve from the thumb piece and provide support for each finger (see p. 145). The fingers and thumb can be flexed fully and the splint enables the hand to grasp and release large objects. It is easily pocketed when not in use.

4. Adherence and contractures of the flexor tendons of the fingers can be stretched by the use of the Capener splint (Fig. 3.56a & b). Commercially-produced wire coil splints, available in different sizes and strengths, are effective in increasing the extension of a slightly flexed proximal interphalangeal joint. The finger can still be flexed actively against the spring wire. Care must be taken in selecting the correct strength for the contractures and the timing, if post-operative, must also be considered.

These splints can also be used to give resistance to weak flexion movements in order to increase strength. The diameter of the wire must be small when used for this purpose.

5. Loss of full finger extension, caused by weakness, contractures and adhesions following surgery, may be corrected by using an outrigger sling (Fig. 3.57); occasionally this may be preferable to any other means of splinting.

Slings round the fingers are attached via elastic bands to spring wire which is welded into a thermoplastic wrist splint. This type of splint is frequently used following Swanson replacement of metacarpophalangeal joints (Swan 1984). It is particularly suited for providing the variation in angle of support for the finger.

An outrigger of Hexcelite provides a simple means to splint one finger. A reinforced extension from the dorsal aspect of the wrist enables one or more rubber bands to be fastened between the outrigger and finger, and can be adjusted for the correct amount of stretch. The angle of pull must always be at 90° to the phalanx.

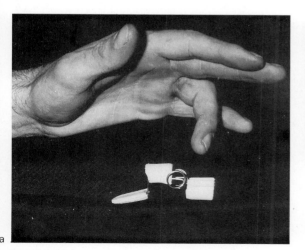 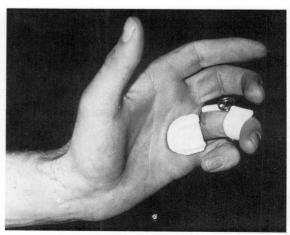

**Fig. 3.56(a & b)** A Capener splint can help to correct a flexion deformity.

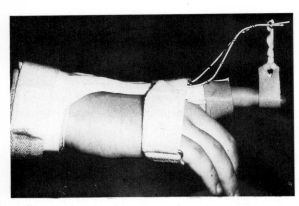

**Fig. 3.57** An outrigger splint may be used to stretch adhesions post-operatively.

Slight stretch only should be given initially as this should be sufficient to correct early post-operative contractures. A persistent contracture will need additional rubber bands to increase the tension.

Loss of finger flexion can be corrected by the pull of rubber bands from the wrist to the finger nails. The bands are attached by hooks glued to the nails. This method has the disadvantage of preventing any normal function while the splint is worn.

### Summary of splinting requirements

The following requirements must be met if splinting is to be successful.
1. The patient must understand the aims and be prepared to co-operate.

2. An effective result must be observed and recorded, otherwise splinting should not be used.
4. The cosmetic appearance of the splint must be acceptable, otherwise the patient will not wear it.
5. The splint must be easy to apply, easy to clean and comfortable to wear.

## HOME PROGRAMME

Although full-time or part-time rehabilitation may be desirable it is not always available, or it may be impossible because of home or occupational problems. When this is the case it is essential that patients understand the need to continue their treatment at home for themselves, not only during the week but at weekends also. Patients should never be allowed to develop the philosophy that treatment ends when they leave the ward, the department or the rehabilitation unit.

Experience has shown also that patients quickly forget the exercises and activities that they are meant to practise. A list of these should therefore be given to each patient to take home as an essential requisite to ensure that nothing will be forgotten. It is most important that activities of daily living are attempted as normally and frequently as possible. Leisure activities play a vital role also and function will be maximised best by both the deliberate and the automatic use of the hand.

## REFERENCES

Barclay V, Collier R J, Jones A 1983 Treatment of various hand injuries by pulsed electromagnetic energy (diapulse). Physiotherapy 69: 9
Capener N 1967 Lively splints. Physiotherapy 53: 11
Dyson M, Suckling J 1978 Stimulation of tissue repair by ultrasound – A survey of the mechanisms involved. Physiotherapy 64: 4
Evans P 1980 The healing process at cellular level: a review. Physiotherapy 66: 8
Frampton V M 1981 Pain control with the aid of transcutaneous nerve stimulation. Physiotherapy 68: 3
Gifford D 1974 Silicone oil for hand trauma. Physiotherapy 60: 11
Kaltenborn F M 1980 Mobilisation of the extremity joints. Olaf Norlis, Oslo
Kleinert H E, Kutz J E, Atasoy E A, Stormo A 1973 Primary repair of flexor tendons. Orthopaedic clinics of North America 4(4)

Knott M, Voss D E 1968 Proprioceptive neuromuscular facilitation. Ballière, Tindall & Cassell, London
Lewith G T, N R 1980 Electrode placement for transcutaneous electrical nerve stimulation (TNS). A method based on classical body acupuncture. R D G Electro-Medical, Croydon
Lipton S 1979 The control of chronic pain, No 2, Current topics in anaesthesia, eds Feldman, Scur. Arnold, London
Maitland G D 1977 Peripheral manipulation. Butterworths, London
Malick M 1979 Manual on static hand splinting. Camp Ltd, Winchester
Melzack R, Wall P D 1965 Pain mechanisms. A new theory. Science 150
Patrick M K 1978 Applications of therapeutic ultrasound. Physiotherapy 64: 4
Raji A R M, Bowden R E M 1983 Effects of high-peak pulsed

electromagnetic field on the degeneration and regeneration of the common peroneal nerve in rats. Journal of Bone and Joint Surgery 65B : 478

Roberts M, Rutherford J H, Harris D 1982 The effect of ultrasound on flexor tendon repairs in the rabbit. The Hand 14: 1

Sherrington C S 1961 The integrative action of the nervous system. Yale University, New Haven

Swan D 1984 Low temperature hand splinting with thermoplastic materials. Physiotherapy 70: 9

Wall P D 1985 The discovery of transcutaneous electrical nerve stimulation. Physiotherapy 71: 8

Wilson D H, Jagerdeesh P 1976 Experimental regeneration in peripheral nerves and the spinal cord in laboratory animals exposed to a pulsed electromagnetic field. Paraplegia 14

Wynn Parry C B 1981 Rehabilitation of the hand. Butterworths, London

# FURTHER READING

Barr N R 1975 The hand. Principles and techniques of simple splintmaking in rehabilitation. Butterworths, London

Cannon N M, Foltz R W, Koepfer J M, Lauck M F, Simpson D M, Bromley R S 1985 Manual of hand splinting. Churchill Livingstone, Edinburgh

Fess E E, Gettle K S, Stickland J W 1981 Hand splinting. Mosby, St Louis, Mo.

Malick M H 1978 Manual on dynamic hand splinting with thermoplastic materials. Camp, Winchester

Melzack R, Wall P D 1983 The challenge of pain. Penguin, Harmondsworth

Wall P D 1984 The painful consequence of peripheral injury Journal of Hand Surgery 9B: 1

Wynn Parry C B 1984 Symposium on pain. Journal of Hand Surgery 9B: 1

# 4

# Traumatic injuries

The injuries and conditions mentioned in this chapter are discussed as separate lesions. It is highly likely when trauma is experienced, however, that damage will have occurred in more than one type of tissue and these additional factors will therefore complicate both assessment and treatment. An attempt has been made to identify the problems and outline the treatment of lesions both in isolation and collectively.

Assessments and treatments have already been discussed in detail in the previous chapters. A description will be given of the signs and symptoms which need assessment, with a brief outline only of the treatment aims and their priorities, together with a rationale of the rehabilitation of these injuries and conditions.

Although dates are given for commencing treatment, it must be realised that these are not always applicable. Some surgeons may agree to earlier treatment than others. The severity of injury and complications during both surgery and recovery will have a bearing on the most suitable day to commence physiotherapy.

Some therapists find themselves supervising and treating patients whose surgery and early postoperative physiotherapy has been carried out in specialised centres. Instructions on this later management should always accompany the patient, but particular queries or worries concerning the patient's treatment can nearly always be answered if a phone call is made direct to the therapist involved.

# FRACTURES

Crucial factors affecting the recovery of function after fractures are the severity and position of the fracture and the duration and position of immobilisation. A fracture into the joint is likely to limit the movement and lead to arthritis in later years.

Immobilisation should be as brief as is necessary to achieve bony union, and the joints should preferably be immobilised either in the 'safe' close-packed position, or in the 'position of function'. If a fracture requires positioning in plaster in a non-functional position it would be better to fix it internally by operation (Semple 1979).

The injury will be accompanied by some degree of soft tissue damage with release of fibrinogen into the surrounding tissues. It is therefore important to reduce any oedema as quickly as possible to prevent permanent fibrosis from occurring, and the hand must therefore be supported in elevation initially.

## Physiotherapy

Early advice from a physiotherapist at a fracture clinic can help the patient to avoid problems which might arise due to his ignorance of his condition. He needs instruction on what should and should not occur, and what he is expected to do with his hand following injury. He must be taught how to exercise his proximal joints to prevent them stiffening, as this can occur very quickly in the elderly. He must also be shown how to exercise the fingers and thumb, if these joints are not splinted, to maintain their mobility. A written list of exercises will help the patient at home, but a check within a week as an out-patient is essential. Often patients are confused following an accident and cannot adequately remember what they have been told to do. Any oedema that may have occurred can be treated immediately, using PEMF and elevated exercises.

When the plaster is removed a crêpe bandage or Tubigrip should be applied to prevent the hand and wrist from swelling. If necessary the arm should be supported in a sling for the first few days.

Ice dips or contrast baths are found to be most effective in returning the circulation to normal after immobilisation in plaster. Wax which produces a vasodilatation of the capillaries is not desirable at this stage as it tends to increase the swelling. A warm water soak, using an arm bath, is an alternative in which the patient actively performs hand movements, squeezing either a ball or shaped forms of Plastazote. Any dead skin can be removed after the soak and hydrous ointment applied if necessary.

Ice may be useful also for its analgesic effect prior to other treatments. If pain is a problem during mobilising sessions the use of TNS can be very effective in allowing the range to be regained more rapidly.

## FRACTURES OF THE WRIST

Injuries occur most commonly from falling onto the outstretched hand, and fractures of the radius and ulna will need up to 6 weeks immobilisation As extension usually proves more difficult to regain than flexion it is preferable for the wrist to be immobilised in a slightly extended position. The plaster should always permit full flexion of the MCP joints.

Severe crushing injuries can cause disruption of the carpus but otherwise fractures of these bones, with the exception of the scaphoid, occur infrequently. When pain continues in the area of the anatomical snuff-box, but a fracture has not initially been diagnosed, the patient should be referred to an orthopaedic consultant. Not all scaphoid fractures can be seen on the first X-ray, and a further examination is therefore essential. A fracture of the proximal pole will need 3 months immobilisation, due to the resulting poor circulation of this section of the bone.

*Physiotherapy* involving supervision and sessions of treatment must be available until good function is achieved. A check-up during the first few days will ensure that the plaster is not becoming too tight. Any report by the patient of tingling must be investigated immediately.

Difficulty may be experienced when the patient is attempting to regain full movement of the wrist and particularly any loss of extension. This is most likely due to the fact that the small gliding movements at the intercarpal and carpometacarpal joints are responsible for a high proportion of wrist extension. These joints, if stiff, are difficult to mobilise unless individual accessory movements are given. The capitate should be identified and all gliding motions given while the wrist is flexed, i.e. when it is in the loose-packed position. Therefore careful assessment of joint range, and especially of the intercarpal joints, should be made. If the patient finds movement painful it is quite probable that the exact position of this pain can be located on examination of the passive physiological and accessory movements, using Kaltenborn's 10 wrist movement plan. Gentle mobilisation of the joint into its painful range will usually, after a few sessions, totally relieve that pain, and the range of wrist movement will then increase automatically. The use of TNS can be of value in reducing pain and discomfort and thereby allowing the mobilisation techniques to be performed efficiently.

Active exercises and functional movements must also be given, increasing the resistance to improve power as quickly as possible. Occupational therapy is of enormous benefit. If it is not available the physiotherapist should ensure that all activities of daily living are possible and that the requirements for employment are ascertained. The patient should attend daily for treatment, if necessary, until it is certain that steady recovery is being made, and that pain-free movement is achieved. Sessions should then be reduced until treatment can be totally ceased. A review is desirable over the next few months to ensure that the progress has been maintained.

During icy conditions in winter many patients are likely to sustain Colles' fractures. This can put considerable strain on the physiotherapy department and may necessitate the use of classes to ensure that some physiotherapy is available for all. It is essential that each patient is assessed initially and that progress is re-evaluated regularly. A certain amount of group activity is excellent, but any particular problems such as persistent oedema, pain and joint stiffness must be treated individually otherwise a satisfactory result will not be achieved.

**Complications**

Reflex sympathetic dystrophy, otherwise known as algodystrophy or Sudeck's atrophy, may occasionally result following a Colles' fracture. Immobilisation

whenever possible in slight wrist extension, prevention of oedema and adequate instruction on the immediate use of the hand followed by regular checks, will usually help to prevent this troublesome condition from occurring. Physiotherapy is essential to remedy any autonomic changes that may appear (see p. 136). Immobilisation should be for as short a time as possible if signs of dystrophy do appear so that intensive treatment may be given.

FRACTURES OF THE METACARPALS AND PHALANGES

Semple (1979) states that most fractures of metacarpals and the distal part of the fingers heal with minimum treatment and few complications. He points to a problem zone, however, of metacarpal head, proximal phalanx and base of the middle phalanx. Any fracture in this area must be diagnosed and treated by a specialist in orthopaedic medicine otherwise deformity will occur, due to the pull of muscles and tendons causing displacement at the fracture site. These fractures may need internal fixation.

A fracture of the shaft of one metacarpal will be splinted by its neighbours and will usually cause little problem. A fracture of the neck of the metacarpal, however, may produce an anterior angulation causing difficulty for correct tendon function and an illusion of joint stiffness. This will require reduction and immobilisation for 2–3 weeks. Fractures of several metacarpals are likely to be accompanied by soft tissue damage, with resulting stiffness of the hand unless it is treated intensively and as early as possible.

Fractures of the proximal phalanx, if not internally fixed, are easily displaced by the pull of the muscles, and therefore need careful immobilisation for a couple of weeks before active treatment commences. The immobilisation of a finger in the flexed position should be avoided. Full extension, or very slight flexion, of the interphalangeal joints with the metacarpophalangeal joints either left free or flexed in approximately 75° of flexion provides a position of function. This allows the patient to use his thumb and available fingers while in the splint and facilitates the later mobilisation of the joints.

Plaster of Paris or thermoplastic materials can be used to make a comfortable splint which, in order to immobilise fractures of the phalanges, should include either one or two neighbour fingers. These are then strapped together, thus providing a stable support. Metal finger splints are less comfortable and rather cumbersome. Cylinders for the fracture of a finger should be avoided.

*Physiotherapy* for simple stable fractures of the metacarpals and phalanges can be introduced when the pain and swelling disappear, usually within 5–7 days of injury. Unstable or compound fractures, and those involving dislocations, may require 3 weeks immobilisation (Fig. 4.1). A crepe bandage, or, for the fingers, a double tubigrip finger stall, may be useful temporarily to prevent swelling and provide a feeling of support in the early treatment stage when free active movements are given.

Mobilisation of the joints by passive physiological and resisted movements should only be commenced when the fractures are united. Passive stretching of joints should never be performed when the articular structures have been involved.

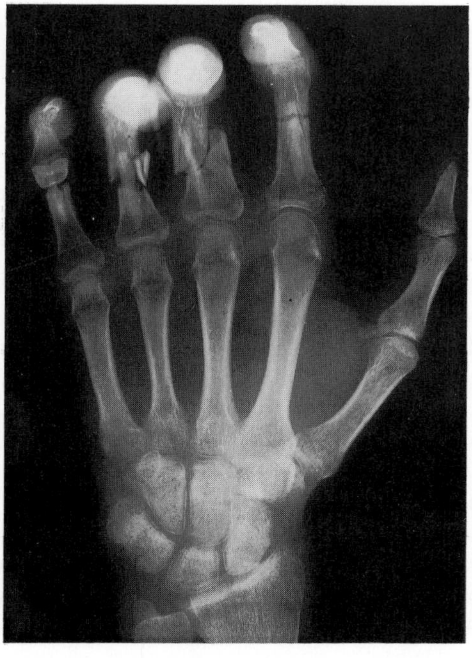

**Fig. 4.1** Unstable or compound fractures may require three weeks immobilisation. This X-ray shows signs of osteoporosis caused by disuse of the hand.

Active exercises, increasing the resistance gradually, will usually achieve a functional result.

MALLET FINGER

Stubbing of the finger tip happens frequently during games such as basketball and volley ball, and occasionally during bed-making, when the extended finger is forcibly flexed, rupturing the extensor mechanism at the distal interphalangeal joint and pulling off a fragment of the terminal phalanx. This prevents active extension of the joint, with the result that the finger tip falls into a flexed position (Fig. 4.2a). Prompt diagnosis and treatment is essential, and immobilisation in a hyperextended position in a cylinder is necessary for up to six weeks (Fig. 4.2b). A commercial metal splint is also available for this purpose. The patient must understand that he should never allow the tip to flex during this time. Gentle mobilising to regain flexion is commenced after six weeks (Fig. 4.2c & d).

## DISLOCATIONS AND JOINT INJURIES

The extent of ligamentous damage together with possible fracture involvement, particularly of the articular surfaces, governs the immediate treatment and length of immobilisation after dislocation. An accurate diagnosis is therefore an essential requirement to ensure a good result. A simple dislocation of an interphalangeal joint, for example, which when reduced is found to be perfectly stable, will need only a short period of rest for 3–4 days, followed by early mobilisation. A dislocation with gross ligamentous damage, however, may need either longer immobilisation in a splint or internal fixation.

### Physiotherapy

The aims of treatment for all dislocations include reduction of oedema and promotion of healing, maintenance of those joints that are free during any immobilisation period, and gentle active rehabilitation as early as possible. Sufficient rest must be given for 3–4 days initially in order to fa-

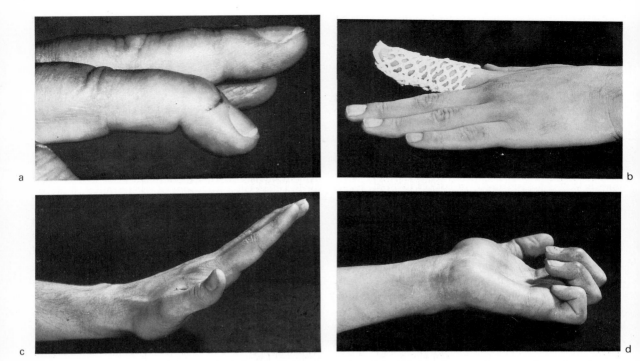

**Fig. 4.2** (a) A mallet finger deformity. (b) Splinted with hyperextension of the DIP joint for 6 weeks. (c) & (d) Final result of extension and flexion.

cilitate the process of repair. The effects of the position in which the hand and wrist are immobilised must be reviewed frequently, and the hand should be kept elevated by a sling for a few days. Ice treatment and PEMF will assist in the reduction of oedema and so should be commenced immediately following injury.

After the initial rest period is over the available joint range should be measured and monitored frequently until treatment is completed. Ice dips are found to be particularly helpful prior to the mobilising sessions as they help to reduce oedema and have a slightly analgesic effect. Wax baths are not suitable as they tend to make the joints swell. Active movements given in warm but not hot water may be preferable if the patient cannot tolerate the cold.

Active, but not passive, physiological movements should be commenced gradually. Resistance should be added only when the range improves and the pain allows. Accessory movements and passive stretching are found to exacerbate both pain and swelling and are therefore contraindicated in the early stages. Slow improvement can usually be gained in all but the most severe injuries by the gradual increase of the patient's own muscle power. The introduction of stronger functional work is therefore a normal progression.

A perilunate dislocation, usually caused by falling onto the hand, displaces the lunate in an anterior direction. It will need surgery to reduce and maintain the bone in correct alignment; otherwise it may press on the median nerve and even cause circulatory damage. The rest of the hand must be kept mobile and intensive treatment given when the wires are removed after 3–4 weeks.

Dislocation of all the carpometacarpal joints may prove unstable when reduced unless pinned and immobilised for 3–4 weeks. It is extremely important during this immobilisation period that the metacarpophalangeal and interphalangeal joints are exercised through as full a range as possible. If the MCP joints have to be immobilised they should be positioned in flexion, if this is at all possible. They will take many weeks of intensive treatment to mobilise if left in extension following this injury.

Dislocation of the metacarpophalangeal and interphalangeal joints, particularly of the latter, occur frequently during games such as cricket, basketball and volley ball. The joints should be examined carefully and diagnosed for bony or ligamentous damage. The possibility of a volar plate rupture should be considered and X-rays taken to exclude its existence. Normal oblique pictures may not show a very small fragment of displaced bone, and true lateral views must therefore be taken. Both collateral ligament and volar plate damage should preferably be repaired immediately by surgical means.

A metacarpophalangeal joint, if stable after reduction, should be rested alongside its neighbours in about 60° flexion with the interphalangeal joints in nearly full extension.

An interphalangeal joint, when stable after reduction, should be rested in nearly full extension beside its neighbours. A plaster of Paris or thermoplastic splint, made individually for two fingers and strapped on, is a more comfortable form of immobilisation than a commercial splint. 3—4 days rest should be adequate for these joints before gentle active mobilisation is commenced. At this stage a double or treble finger stall made of double thickness Tubigrip helps to prevent oedema, and the neighbour fingers provide lateral support during movements.

When a volar plate injury is suspected but has not been repaired, it is essential to immobilise the joint in flexion for 2—3 weeks to allow the rupture to heal. Following this the joint should be mobilised very gradually into extension. A two part splint of metal pieces, which are bent and fit over the dorsum of the finger, permits full active flexion of the joint but prevents full extension (Fig. 4.3a & b). The splint is easily adjusted by altering the degree of bend in the splint. If there is any residual loss of extension, which cannot be regained either by active or passive stretching, a Capener splint will usually help to stretch the contractures (Fig. 4.3c).

## JOINT DEFORMITIES

Specific deformities in the joints of the hand and wrist occur as the result of joint injury, from an imbalance of muscle control, from rheumatic

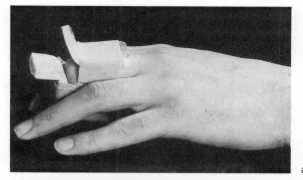
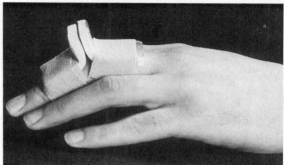
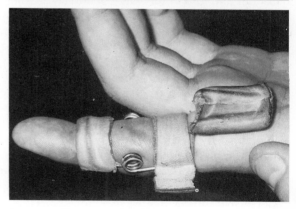

**Fig. 4.3**  Following a volar plate injury: (a) A two-part splint permits active flexion, (b) but limits extension. (c) A Capener splint assists recovery of full PIP joint extension.

disease and from congenital deformities. Fractures which unite in poor alignment may also give the impression of a deformity at a nearby joint and will affect the structures that pass over that joint.

Correct positioning after injury should help to prevent a deformity from either occurring or becoming fixed. Utilising the close-packed position also ensures that the joints are in the best position of function. Fixed deformities that have already

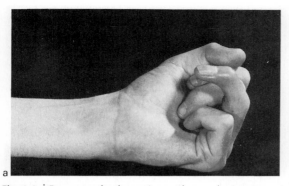 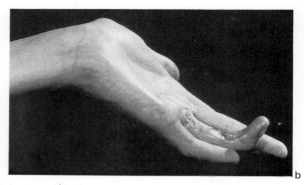

**Fig. 4.4** One year after laceration and several operations and infections of the finger, (a) & (b) show the limitation of movement. Further conservative treatment proved inadequate and the patient requested that finger be amputated.

developed will need intensive treatment to regain both mobility and joint control. If this fails surgery may need to be considered in order to correct the deformity and prevent its recurrence.

Stiffness of one joint, especially of either a metacarpophalangeal joint or a proximal interphalangeal joint, can cause a crippling disability as the finger sticks out and gets in the way continually. If joints of all fingers are similarly affected, even with considerable loss of range as can occur following severe burns of the hand, the disability will in fact not be so great.

A joint replacement may be considered if only the joint itself is affected. As problems caused by trauma often involve other structures also, a replacement is not always suitable and silastic replacements are not usually desirable in fit young men. The patient's own metatarsophalangeal joint may, however, be considered for the replacement of a metacarpophalangeal joint.

Corrective surgery may or may not succeed and will inevitably be time-consuming. In a young active person the quickest way to return function when one finger has become an extreme nuisance may be to amputate (Fig. 4.4a & b). This is a decision that can only be made by the patient after all attempts at rehabilitation have failed. Some patients will think of this remedy for themselves, while others will not consider it at any cost.

## Boutonnière or Buttonhole deformity

This deformity results mainly from trauma to the dorsum of the finger at the level of the proximal interphalangeal joint, when damage is caused to the central slip of the extensor expansion. The lateral slips slide anteriorly and therefore produce a flexion deformity. Attempts at extension fail to gain full extension of the proximal interphalangeal joint but will cause hyperextension at the terminal interphalangeal joint. Due to the altered mechanics of the joints the position of the retinacular ligament is changed and, if allowed, it will contract. The resulting hyperextension contracture at the distal interphalangeal joint thus prevents both active and passive flexion from occurring and the joint quickly stiffens. If this injury is not treated urgently the deformity that results will become extremely difficult to correct.

Direct finger injury and burns are the most common traumatic causes (Fig. 4.5) and will need careful preventative positioning by splinting the proximal interphalangeal joint in full extension for 3–4 weeks, and at the same time allowing active distal joint flexion. A cylinder which terminates immediately proximal to the distal interphalangeal joint or a strong Capener style splint (Fig. 4.3) are both suitable as they maintain the extensor expansion in the central position, allowing it to heal, while the retinacular ligament is held on a stretch. Active movement of both MCP and DIP joints can still be given. If the extensor expansion has been cleanly divided it will need immediate surgery.

After 3 weeks of immobilisation, dynamic splintage is desirable, using a weak Capener splint which allows some active but controlled flexion at the PIP joint. It also maintains extension of the PIP joint at rest, allows flexion of the DIP joint and protects the proximal joint during early mobilisation. Active flexion and extension of the PIP joint should be increased very gradually at this stage. Forced passive flexion must never be given.

A residual boutonnière deformity is difficult to correct conservatively, especially when the joints have become stiff. The finger is vulnerable to knocks, which can result in a painful proximal interphalangeal joint. Surgery at this stage is not usually successful and it is occasionally found that a severely deformed finger may eventually need amputation.

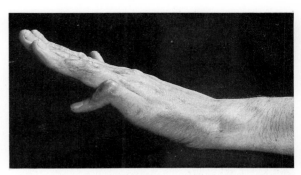

**Fig. 4.5** These Boutonnière deformities in the little finger and mild swan-neck deformity of the ring finger, were caused by burns.

### Swan neck deformity

This deformity, most commonly found with rheumatic disease, can also occur as the result of trauma (Fig. 4.5). There is hyperextension of the proximal interphalangeal joint and flexion at the distal interphalangeal joint. Frequently, the patient has difficulty in initiating active flexion of the PIP joint as the lateral slips of the retinacular ligament slide in a dorsal direction and lie, therefore, on the dorsal side of the fulcrum of the joint. Passive flexion of the PIP joint and passive extention of the DIP joint may both be limited.

Absence or weakness of flexor digitorum superficialis, when combined with normal profundus action, can eventually result in the same deformity, showing a volar prominence together with some hyperextension of the PIP joint, e.g. the long-term effect following a graft of flexor digitorum profundus when superficialis has been excised. One of the roles of FDS, besides its flexor control, is to prevent this hyperextension of the PIP joint.

A swan-neck deformity may also result from an intrinsic contracture when the volar surface of the PIP joint becomes prominent. This is due to the strong inelastic pull of the ischaemic intrinsic muscles which insert into the dorsal expansion immediately distal to the PIP joint.

The deformity is not easy to correct conservatively, especially when it is due to lack of full muscle control. Joint mobility must be regained and the patient taught to perform his exercises for himself. A Capener splint which holds the PIP joint in a few degrees of flexion can sometimes be helpful as the small amount of flexion provided enables active flexion to be initiated correctly at the PIP joint.

## AMPUTATIONS

Direct trauma can cause varying degrees of finger or hand amputation. The resulting disability will depend largely on the site of amputation together with the effects of any other tissue damage. Some patients have the motivation and ability to overcome their problems better than others, and manage to achieve remarkable function despite loss of digits (Fig. 4.6a & b).

Whole hand amputation is a devastating disability for the patient. Activity may be possible to a certain extent by the use of a prosthesis, but sensory function is totally irreplaceable. With the advances of modern surgery replantation is succeeding more frequently. Its main advantage is the retention of some sensation, besides the improved function and cosmetic effect.

### Causes

Causes of amputation include trauma from road or industrial accidents, gunshot wounds and blast injuries. Circular saws are a particularly common cause of accidents to carpenters resulting in loss of part of the hand or fingers. Surgical amputation may become a necessity in older people because of the effects of a circulatory disorder. It may very occasionally be considered the only solution for the total paralysis of a limb or for the residual deformity of a finger. The procedure should be implemented only when all other methods have failed and the patient particularly desires this course of action.

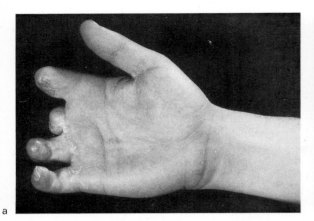

a

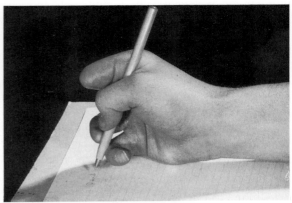

c

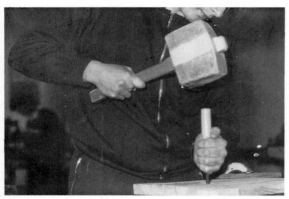

b

**Fig. 4.6(a, b & c)**  Well-motivated patients can achieve remarkable function despite loss of digits.

## Sites of amputation

Loss of the thumb causes incapacitating dysfunction to the hand and it is essential that some pollicisation technique is performed if the amputated thumb cannot be replanted. In multiple amputation of digits, including the thumb, it may be possible to replant one of the amputated fingers in the thumb position. Later a great or second toe, or alternatively a ring or index finger, may be pollicised. Usually a digit from the same hand is transposed together with its neurovascular supply. Therefore, not only will the hand need retraining in movement but the location of sensation will need intensive re-education also.

Amputation of the index finger alone is not severely disabling in most cases because the middle finger has the ability to replace index function. Hand activity can be effectively retained when the patient has a normal thumb remaining unless he practises such skills as typing or piano playing.

Amputation of several fingers will inevitably produce a far more serious disability, as the greater the number of amputated digits the greater will be the loss of function. Little finger amputation may cause difficulty to those persons who need to use the dynamic tripod position, i.e. for writing, painting or other delicate and precise movements with the hands, as the little finger normally supports the hand during this activity.

For those needing power grasp it is better that a portion of the finger is retained, amputating, if it becomes a necessity, immediately proximal to the head of the proximal phalanx. Cosmetically this is not so noticeable as may be anticipated, as the fingers usually rest in the flexed position and the loss of the distal part of the finger is therefore not too obvious. For women who are very concerned

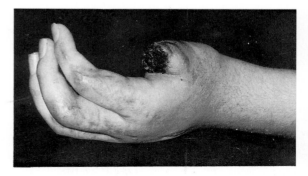

**Fig. 4.7**  Amputation of the thumb causes enormous physical and psychological dysfunction. It is essential that a pollicisation is performed if replantation cannot be performed.

about the cosmetic effect, the amputation of index or little finger may be shaped obliquely, immediately proximal to the head of the metacarpal. Removal by filletting of the whole of the metacarpal of middle or ring fingers, and the subsequent closing-in of any residual gap, will leave a slightly weakened but cosmetically improved hand. The residual disability of this procedure, especially in the early post-operative weeks, is for coins and small objects to slip through the gap between the fingers.

## Physiotherapy

A straightforward traumatic or surgical amputation should heal quickly and need relatively little early physiotherapy. However, amputations as the result of blast, crush injuries or gunshot wounds, with their extensive soft tissue damage, will need far more intensive treatment to ensure maximum mobility of the hand, as described under the treatment of crush injuries.

The hand and arm must be elevated to reduce oedema, whatever the extent of the amputation and whether the patient is in bed or ambulant. Adjacent joints should be kept mobile by gentle, active and, if necessary, assisted movements, usually commenced the day following surgery. Early movements should be given to increase range of the joints towards the 'safe' position in particular. Tendon activity should be aimed primarily at regaining flexion of the fingers, before extension is achieved.

Psychologically, and especially initially, the loss of fingers or part or whole of the hand can be very traumatic, and for some time the patient will probably suffer a degree of shock. A sympathetic but increasingly positive approach should be made by the therapist, by pointing out the ability of the hand to adapt to the situation. Photographs which demonstrate the function other patients have achieved are enormously useful at this stage. Function can become remarkably efficient, even with the loss of fingers, when the patient makes a determined effort to overcome his disability.

Tenderness of the stump is likely to be experienced following the amputation. As the healing continues and the stump settles an increase in contact between stump and objects must be encour-

aged, commencing with handling and gentle tapping by the physiotherapist's fingers. It must be ensured that the patient actually uses the end of his stump, as the sensory input will help to lessen any tender or painful sensations. The tenderness will be worse with a poor suture line, particularly when it is badly positioned, and also if the amputated nerve ends become tethered to skin, bone or underlying tissue. Adhesions should be loosened by massage, and TNS used for reducing any pain and discomfort whilst also allowing the patient to use his stump more freely.

Phantom awareness is another symptom which most patients experience following amputation. Only a small proportion, however, will suffer phantom pain for long (5 to 10%), when it may either be continual or spasmodic. It is likely to be more severe if the hand or finger could not be saved due to the extent of primary injury. If the patient suffers pain prior to amputation the pain patterns may continue as phantom pain after surgery. Established pain should therefore be eliminated if at all possible prior to an amputation.

TNS is effective in curing long-standing phantom limb pain, and can also be used to prevent that pain from occurring. It should be commenced the day following operation to inhibit the establishment of pain patterns. The electrodes should be placed over the appropriate nerve trunk, and the optimum position may be discovered by changing the position of the electrodes during the first few days. Accurate records of positioning must therefore be kept.

Distraction by becoming absorbed in some occupation is one of the best ways of forgetting pain, and this is of particular relevance for those suffering from phantom pain. The advantage of having a good occupational therapy department for the patient with this type of problem cannot be stressed too strongly.

Temporary prostheses made in the workshops or occupational therapy departments can improve function considerably and need not be complicated. For example, a prosthesis to provide extra length to a shortened digit can make a required activity, such as typing, possible. It is a great advantage if the patient himself helps to design and work on his own prosthesis. Fibre glass is a useful material which can be fastened to the patient with leather and velcro fastenings. Attachments for holding tools can be fixed into the fibre glass, which can be drilled for this purpose.

A prosthesis must be requested from the nearest limb fitting centre for the loss of the whole hand. Adequate training in its use and suitable attachments will be made available at the centre. Cosmetic hands and fingers with excellent shape and likeness to the normal hand, are also available from the limb fitting centres. These must be offered to the patient, as appearing in public with an obvious amputation is psychologically traumatic to most people. Further aspects on the psychological problems of patients with hand injuries can be found in Chapter 2.

## Replantation

With the advance of surgery following the widespread use of the microscope in the theatre it is possible on occasion to replant an amputated limb or digit. This depends almost entirely on the ability of the surgeon to restore an adequate circulation quickly enough to ensure viability of the tissues. After an accident a limb or digit should be placed immediately in a polythene bag and the bag put into a container with crushed ice in order to slow the metabolic rate and allow a greater delay between the amputation and replantation.

Bones must be immobilised, and sufficient skin coverage given to prevent loss of fluid and also infection. By preference nerves should be sutured immediately, but these may have to be left, together with any divided tendons, for later surgery.

The aims of treatment for the physiotherapist are to prevent oedema, to assist the venous return, and to maintain the mobility of any joints that are freely available. The joints immediately proximal and distal to the site of the injury may have been immobilised in order to allow bony union to take place. Never, for at least 3–4 weeks, must the movements place any strain on sutured or grafted arteries and veins as this could jeopardise the circulation to the limb which has been so carefully restored. The physiotherapist must be quite sure that the treatments given are with the full agreement of the surgeon in charge of the case.

Distal joints, even though the patient cannot move them himself due to division of muscles,

tendons and nerves, must be regularly exercised passively by the physiotherapist and later, with instruction, by the patient himself. Joints must be kept mobile, even at the expense of sutured nerves and tendons. The pumping action of the joints is also a means by which the oedema will be reduced, besides maintaining mobility. Out-rigger splintage, utilising any available antagonist or prime mover function is helpful in retaining mobility.

The later physiotherapy will need to be intensive, with full-time rehabilitation a necessity. Treatment will depend on the assessments, together with the analysis of the problems. These will probably include stiff joints, severe adherence at the site of amputation, paralysis of muscles, sensory loss, and poor circulation. The return of useful function will prove a challenge to the therapists.

## Complications

The main complications after amputation, besides the loss of function, usually concern the severence of peripheral nerves. The axons, following the initial Wallerian degeneration, commence to sprout in an attempt to discover their endoneurial tubes. With the distal nerve amputated their search is abortive, with the result that they turn in many directions, forming a demyelinated neuroma.

Most neuromata are non-symptomatic, but any problems will depend mainly on local factors. Gross scarring with contracting fibrous tissue formation is considered the most likely cause of a troublesome neuroma. Careful resection of the nerve at the time of amputation and provision of the nerve end with a good tissue bed is the best prevention of later symptoms. Surgery, with transportation of the nerve to an adjacent site that is free of scarring and less liable to trauma is sometimes undertaken but the results have proved extremely disappointing.

Gentle tapping at first in an area surrounding the neuroma and gradually approaching the tender spot until right over it, will frequently improve and occasionally relieve all painful symptoms. The patient should be shown how to continue the tapping for himself, as an ongoing treatment may be needed. A vibrator provides a gentle method of commencing this treatment in extremely painful cases and the use of TNS may allow the therapist

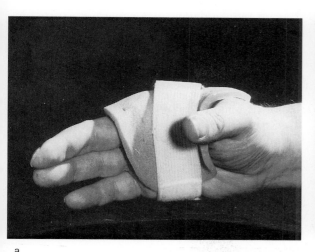

a

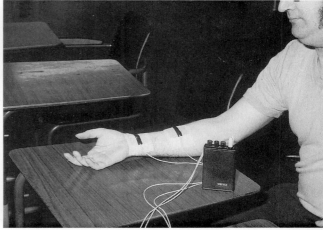

b

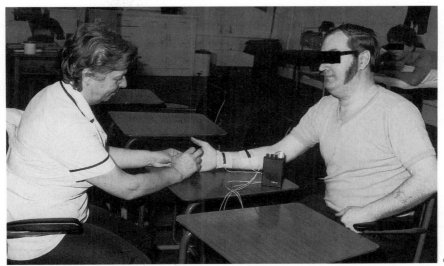

c

**Fig. 4.8** (a) Amputation of index finger. (b) TNS can effectively reduce the discomfort of neuromata and (c) can allow the therapist to handle and perform the tapping more comfortably.

to perform the vibration or tapping more comfortably (Fig. 4.8b & c). It should be used during several hours of the day, with the electrodes sited over the section of the nerve proximal to its neuroma. The patient must be encouraged to use his amputated stump as normally as possible as pain may increase if there is inadequate sensory input to the affected area. A padded splint or leather cuff may be effective in protecting a painful neuroma (Fig. 4.8a).

Extremely tender or hyperpathic areas adjacent to the line of incision may produce severe stump pain. TNS and pressure splinting using Plastazote or elasticated garments can help to reduce this problem by the input of normal sensory stimuli and utilisation of the pain-gate theory. Revision of the stump may eventually have to be considered.

Severe and long-standing phantom limb pain can frequently be reduced by the use of TNS. It has been known to completely eliminate phantom pain after fifty years continuous duration. A determined effort must be made by the rehabilitation team not only to reduce the pain but also to return the patient to work as soon as possible. Mental occupation with its increase of central inhibition of the pain pathways is probably the most effective means of phantom pain control.

## CRUSH INJURIES

These injuries are probably the most severely disabling to the hand, mainly due to the resulting fibrosis of the soft tissues. Every feasible type of complication may be present including:

1. Arterial or venous damage needing anastomosis or graft. A ligation is not a desirable technique but is still frequently practised.
2. Soft tissue damage, requiring excision of any non-viable muscle and skin. The resulting oedema with its release of fibrinogen, can cause extensive fibrosis and stiffness.
3. Fractures and joint disruption, requiring immobilisation.
4. Skin loss and degloving requiring coverage to prevent infection and loss of tissue fluid.
5. Nerve injury needing repair by suture or grafting procedure.
6. Tendon or muscle damage, requiring a primary or secondary repair or graft. Tendon transfers may be necessary later.
7. Amputation, either immediately in extremely severe cases, or later because of developing necrosis.

The most urgent need is to ensure adequate vascularisation as otherwise the viability of the limb or part will be a risk. This is followed by immobilisation of fractures and dislocations and provision of skin coverage.

### Physiotherapy

Active physiotherapy may be difficult in the early days, as the conditions may either necessitate immobilisation following surgery, or have caused immobility by both the division of nerves and tendons and the gross oedema. This oedema must be reduced as quickly as possible as the resulting fibrosis causes the greatest disability by developing into a stiff hand (Fig. 4.9).

Correct positioning into the 'safe' position, with the hand and arm elevated to reduce oedema, is therefore essential. The positioning will ensure that the finger tip and thumb approximation will be functional, even though limitation of other movements may persist. The hand must never be allowed to remain fully extended as it may well become 'frozen' in this position and be totally non-functional.

All methods should be utilised to reduce the oedema and gentle active movements should, whenever possible, be commenced within the first 2–3 days of injury. Closed environmental therapy (CET), which blows sterile air at high pressure into the encompassing plastic bag, can be useful as it allows the hand to move inside the bag. This early active treatment must be agreed with the surgeon initially. Pulsed electromagnetic fields (PEMF) should be used when available as they can be given through dressings and even plaster of Paris, and are effective in reducing fibrosis and assisting the healing process. Ice and ultrasonics can also be used on accessible areas of the skin.

Silicone oil, sterilised and contained in a large jar, provides a particularly useful medium for early exercising of crush injuries. It is comfortable for the patient, allows debris to drop off the skin and

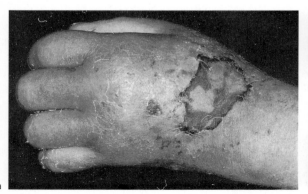
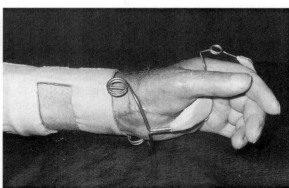

**Fig. 4.9** (a) A crush injury showing severe oedema. (b) Dynamic splint aimed to improve wrist extension and MCP joint flexion.

appears to hasten the healing process. In particular it encourages the patient to exercise his joints actively and when necessary the physiotherapist can move the joints through a passive range. The container must be of a really large size for this to be done.

The intensity of treatment should be increased as quickly as possible during the first few weeks and full-time rehabilitation instituted if a stiff hand is developing. Pneumotherapy will help to reduce the oedema when the skin is healed, and massage and all active and passive treatments including accessory movements should be given with the hand in an elevated position. Treatment should continue throughout the day if a satisfactory result is to be achieved.

Passive stretching is necessary when the range remains limited and particularly when active movement is still not possible. Initially the stretch should be applied gently and gradually. A strong stretch

must be delayed until seven or eight weeks after injury, otherwise an exacerbation of fibrosis will result. Stretch splinting, following the physiotherapist's manual stretch may then be introduced. Sansplint XR or plaster of Paris are suitable material to use. The patient should wear a stretch splint at lunch-time and a resting splint at night.

Thumb and finger webs are liable to contract and will need active and passive stretching to prevent or correct any deformity. Wedge splints will help to maintain a stretch of the webs if applied during the lunch-time, together with a resting wedge splint worn at night. Polyform and Polyflex are the most suitable materials for this purpose, as they conform exactly to the contours of the webs.

The priority in the plan to provide maximum hand function is to regain joint range in the following order:

1. Full metacarpophalangeal joint flexion (Fig. 4.10a & b) and simultaneous interphalangeal

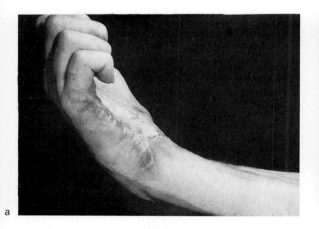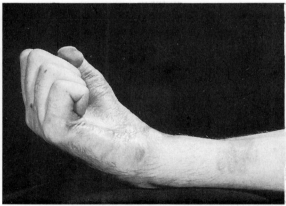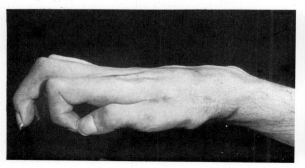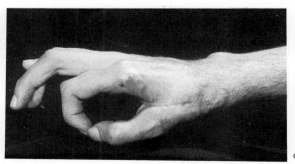

**Fig. 4.10** (a) A crush injury with limited MCP flexion. (b) With improvement after several weeks treatment. (c) Extremely limited thumb function. (d) Improved after resection of fibrosis and an opponens transfer.

joint extension together with palmar abduction of the thumb, will ensure finger to thumb tip function and lateral pinch.

2. Flexion of the interphalangeal joints to give flexion of finger tips to palm, thus providing grasp.

3. Full and simultaneous extension of all the metacarpophalangeal and interphalangeal joints ensuring the ability to stretch the fingers to grasp round and release an object.

4. Extension and ulnar deviation together with pronation and supination are the more essential movements of the wrist which should be re-gained concurrently with movements of the fingers and thumb.

Range should be constantly monitored to ensure that a gain in one direction is not made at the expense of a loss in another. Passive range of joints is the most essential function. If active movement does not recover there are usually surgical pro-cedures to consider later which might return some function to the hand (Fig. 4.10c & d).

Severe crush injuries are likely to need several weeks or months of intensive treatment and even then some are extremely unlikely to recover fully. Short-session treatments, though daily, cannot achieve a good functional result, as by the time the patient has arrived home his hand condition is usually back to where it started that morning. Full-time treatment in a rehabilitation unit is most likely to achieve the best functional result for the patient.

## ISCHAEMIC CONTRACTURES

These contractures, which result from vascular impairment, may be caused by road traffic acci-dents, industrial injuries and gunshot wounds. A fairly common cause also is from tight plasters which, if not removed quickly, constrict the arterial flow, resulting in damage to the muscles and oc-casionally to the nerves and skin also.

A contracture may not on initial observation be instantly obvious, but nevertheless it can be severely disabling to the patient. The normal func-tion of the hand, especially when intricate move-ments are involved, can only be achieved by the combined action of the long extrinsic and small intrinsic muscles. Ischaemia can cause extensive

fibrosis, when the muscles will be unable either to contract efficiently or extend fully. Moreover there will be an impairment of proprioception, which when the intrinsic muscles are involved is especially disabling.

Volkmann's ischaemic contracture affects the muscles of the forearm, usually the flexors only, but with a severe injury it may involve the extensors also (Fig. 4.11a). Contractures of the long flexors will prevent full and simultaneous extension of the wrist, fingers and thumb. When the wrist is flexed, however, the fingers and thumb will usually be able to extend (Fig. 4.11b). Conversely, as the wrist extends, the contracture of the flexors will passively pull the fingers and thumb into a greater degree of flexion, which is a form of tenodesis action (Fig. 4.11c). Contracture of the extensor muscles will prevent full flexion of wrist, fingers and thumb simultaneously (Fig. 4.11d). The in-volvement of both flexors and extensors will there-fore limit function severely.

Vascular injury at the wrist or in the hand may cause ischaemia, leading to fibrosis of the intrinsic muscles and thus producing an intrinsic contracture. The muscles, when severely contracted, cause the metacarpophalangeal joints to be held in flexion together with the interphalangeal joints in extension (Fig. 4.12a). The reverse of this position, i.e. a combination of MCP joint extension and IP joint flexion will be impossible to achieve, even with a strong passive stretch (Fig. 4.12b). When the thenar muscles are affected the thumb becomes clamped tightly across the palm, close to the fingers (Fig. 4.12c). Virtually no thumb movement may be possible, and moreover the thumb will be in the way of finger flexion which combines to limit hand function almost entirely.

A complication of severe ischaemia may be nerve damage causing motor and sensory loss. The circulation of the hand will be affected therefore by both the direct vascular damage and by the autonomic involvement. It is essential that the patient is thoroughly warned concerning the need to protect his hand and to keep it warm in cold weather.

*Assessment* for contractures should include an observation of the hand and forearm at rest and the affected hand compared with the contra-lateral limb. Particular note should be made of the pos-

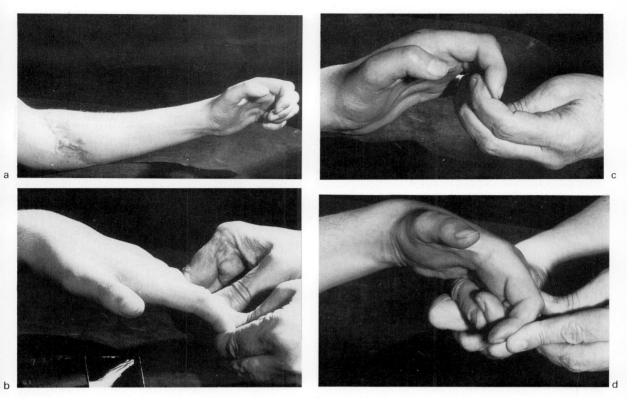

**Fig. 4.11**   (a) A patient with a severe Volkmann's contracture affecting both flexors and extensors. (b) Passive extension of fingers achieved only when wrist was flexed. (c) As the wrist extended the fingers were pulled tightly into flexion. (d) Neither active nor passive flexion of wrist and fingers simultaneously is possible due to the contracture of the extensors.

ition of the fingers and thumb and of both dorsal and volar surfaces of the joints. The following tests should then be performed to identify, or eliminate, the presence of contractures.

1. To identify a contracture of the long flexors the patient is asked to extend wrist, fingers and thumb as far as possible and at the same time. The Salter scale can be used to measure the excursion of movement.

A mild contracture will only prevent movement into full outer range. It may, however, be sufficiently severe that it prevents the muscles from being extended further than mid-range. The physiotherapist should therefore apply over-pressure in order to feel how much the movement is restricted and to eliminate lack of range as a result of muscle weakness or paralysis. The active movement combining wrist, finger and thumb flexion should also be examined. A comparison should be made with the range of the contralateral limb and a note taken of any restriction which may be caused by adherent scars or stiff joints.

2. To identify a contracture of the long extensors the patient is asked to flex his wrist, fingers and thumb at the same time. Over-pressure is then given by the physiotherapist to feel the degree of contracture. The range of wrist flexion is measured when the fingers are flexed. Adherence of scars, weakness of movement and the amount of active extension available should again be tested and compared with the contralateral limbs.

3. To identify a possible intrinsic contracture the patient is asked firstly to flex then extend all the metacarpophalangeal and interphalangeal joints together. A really severe intrinsic contracture will prevent full metacarpophalangeal joint extension, so this movement needs to be tested passively and in isolation by the therapist. The range should be recorded. Secondly, the patient is requested to keep his interphalangeal joints flexed while he

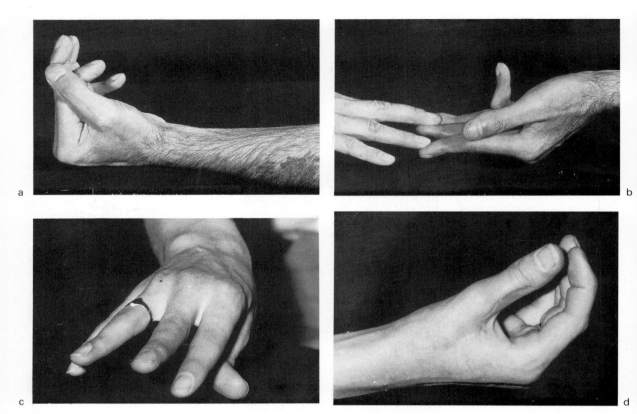

**Fig. 4.12** Typical intrinsic contractures when (a) the patient is unable to flex his IP joints, and (b) extend his MCP joints. (c) Another patient with inability to abduct the fingers and thumb. The thumb position also prevented him from making a fist. (d) The 'claw' position should be attempted.

attempts to extend his metacarpophalangeal joints. Over-pressure should again be given by the physiotherapist to feel the extent of any contracture.

This attempted 'claw' position (Fig. 4.12d) should be demonstrated to the patient initially and tried with his normal hand. Observation should again be made that scars are not adherent, and that joints have not become stiff, thus preventing the required movement.

4. To identify thenar muscle contractures the patient is asked to first extend and then abduct his thumb as fully as possible. The therapist should also apply over-pressure in order to test these movements passively.

## Physiotherapy

Scarring from the injury may have impaired the venous and lymphatic return; therefore early attention will be needed to reduce any resulting oedema.

Scars when soundly healed, should be given a stretching massage using lanolin as the medium. Exercise with its pumping action should then follow. All treatments should be given in elevation when oedema is present.

Contractures of the forearm flexors should be stretched, the therapist gradually increasing and sustaining the pull on the muscles and at the same time watching the effect on the patient. The physiotherapist should apply the stretch with one hand whilst supporting the mobile joints with the other to prevent any hyperextension. This procedure will probably be uncomfortable but should never be so extreme that it is painful. The movements should never be jerky as they might cause further damage to the fibrosed muscle fibres. During the subsequent weeks of treatment the aim is to achieve full and simultaneous extension of the wrist and fingers.

Active exercises follow the stretch regime; the patient must be able to actively maintain the increased range obtained passively by the therapist. If the long flexor muscles have become extremely contracted it is the extensors especially which will need strengthening. PNF techniques are a suitable means by which to achieve both lengthening and strengthening effects.

Patients should attend for several sessions a day: if these are held early and late in the morning and again in the afternoon the contractures will be treated with sufficient intensity. After the first morning and afternoon sessions the patient should use his hand functionally to make full use of any gained movement. After the last session a stretch splint should be applied for an hour which will maintain the hand and wrist in the maximum stretched position. The splint should extend from mid-forearm to just beyond the finger tips. At night the patient should wear a splint which maintains a comfortable but optimum position.

For intrinsic contractures the aim is to obtain simultaneous extension of the metacarpophalangeal joints together with flexion of the interphalangeal joints. The stretch towards this claw position of the hand should be applied gradually and be followed by strong active exercise for flexors digitorum profundus and superficialis. The MCP joints should be held in as much extension as possible. A palmar splint which extends distally just beyond the MCP joints but not as far as the proximal interphalangeal joints, will allow the IP joints to be flexed over the end and be bandaged down firmly (see Fig. 3.52). It may also be used when exercising the long flexors of the fingers.

Because the intrinsic muscles are so small they are less likely to respond to the stretching procedures than the forearm muscles. Any residual and disabling contractures of either long flexors or intrinsics may need a surgical release and tendon transfer procedure to improve hand function.

## DUPUYTREN'S CONTRACTURE

Dupuytren's contracture is a relatively common condition in the Anglo-Saxon race (McCallum & Hueston 1962), especially in those over the age of 65, and occurs ten times more frequently in men than in women. It is a disorder of collagen, when the fascia underlying the skin becomes thickened and fibrotic, but the cause of the condition remains unknown. The fascia later contracts, thereby causing a flexion deformity to develop in the fingers and occasionally in the thumb.

Physiotherapy plays a relatively limited role in conservative management of this condition. The maximum joint range may be preserved for some time by teaching the patient how to stretch his own contractures and by the application of a stretch splint, but in no way can this treatment prevent the eventual advance of the disease. It is essential therefore that the patient should consult an experienced surgeon before the joint contractures become irreversible. Muscle power should be maintained to facilitate activity both pre- and post-operatively.

### Post-operative treatment

Following a fasciotomy, when the affected tissue has been resected, a fluffy compression bandage is applied over the dressing and the hand elevated to prevent oedema. Surgical techniques, post-operative management, the positioning and the duration of immobilisation can vary considerably. Usually the hand is placed in as full extension as possible but sometimes the metacarpophalangeal joints are positioned in flexion for a few days with the interphalangeal joints in nearly full extension. Some surgeons prefer the open-palm technique when skin closure is difficult as this allows drainage and prevents the formation of haematomas (McCash 1964). Skin grafting or the transportation of a flap may be necessary: it is found that a recurrence of the disorder rarely occurs directly under the graft (Harrison & Morris 1975).

Exercise must be given to the shoulder and elbow as this will help to maintain both the circulation of the limb and the mobility of the joints. With the agreement of the surgeon, active movement of the hand usually commences 2–3 days after surgery unless skin grafting has been performed. The padding is removed to allow movement, and gentle active extension, in particular, and flexion and abduction exercises are given to the fingers and thumb. Opposition of the thumb towards each individual finger should be gently performed. Special attention must be paid to any oedema which may have occurred. Massage to the fingers and active movements are found to be the most effective treatment to reduce any swelling.

After a few days, when the hand is redressed following exercise, a splint should be applied to position the fingers in the optimum degree of extension that can be held comfortably. Stretch must not be applied at this stage. Treatment should be repeated several times daily, gradually gaining a little more extension, with the splint being altered accordingly.

After 1 week more emphasis is placed on regaining full finger flexion. The stitches are removed on about the 10th day when, if the healing is satisfactory, the tempo of treatment may be increased.

Healing of the scars may be slow, especially if the condition was advanced prior to surgery. Ultrasonics, saline soaks, massage around the area and active movements in silicone oil will all help to stimulate the circulation and improve healing.

After 2-3 weeks any adherent scars should be massaged with lanolin and treated with ultrasound. If the surrounding area is particularly thickened and indurated a small polyform splint, moulded directly to the part, should be bandaged firmly on to the healed scar and skin. When combined with exercise it helps to loosen any structures that might be tethered, as well as softening the scarring and induration.

Webs should be stretched, as they may have become contracted prior to the operation, and stiff joints should be mobilised using accessory and active movements. Very gradual passive stretching may be introduced at 3 weeks, but only if absolutely necessary and after healing has taken place. The use of serial stretch splints may be needed after 4 weeks to restore extension by applying a gentle stretch for several short sessions during the day, and maintaining an optimum but comfortable position at night. An alternative method is to use a dynamic glove which has lengths of clock spring attached over the dorsum of hand and fingers. The glove applies a constant dynamic stretch to the fingers.

## Complications

A finger that was severely contracted down into flexion may suffer some complications from surgery as an excess of stretch on nerves, blood vessels and skin compromises these tissues. Pain with increasing stiffness and swelling must also be watched for carefully. Kleinert et al (1982) reported that 22% of 130 patients who had undergone fasciotomy developed post-traumatic sympathetic dystrophy. This condition must be recognised quickly before it becomes severe, so that it can be treated by TNS and as much movement as possible (see below).

Mild finger deformities may develop following surgery: for example, a swan-neck may result due to the extent of fascia release on the volar aspect of the proximal interphalangeal joint. A small finger splint such as a Capener, which prevents full PIP joint extension, will usually correct this problem.

## REFLEX SYMPATHETIC DYSTROPHY

This condition, known also as Sudeck's atrophy and algodystrophy, can result in a severe problem that is often far worse than the initial injury itself. Why it occurs in some people yet not in others is still not fully understood, and studies by psychologists have shown no consistent pattern of personality involvement. What is absolutely certain is that it must be treated instantly and urgently in order to prevent it from becoming an acute problem that is difficult to cure.

The dystrophy usually follows a comparatively minor injury, i.e. a sprain, a Colles' fracture, soft tissue injury and surgery, e.g. a fasciotomy for a Dupuytren's contracture. It follows crush injuries and peripheral nerve involvement less frequently.

The main signs and symptoms include:
1. Oedema
2. Pain which is far more severe than can be anticipated for the underlying condition
3. Excessive sweating at first
4. Colour and temperature changes
5. Osteoporosis shown on X-ray
6. Unwillingness to move the hand.

At first the hand becomes hot and swollen with pronounced sweating. The patient will probably dislike both using his hand and having it touched. These signs and symptoms worsen if the condition is not treated, becoming more acutely painful in particular. There may be two kinds of pain: a spontaneous burning pain and hyperpathia, the acutely painful response to touch.

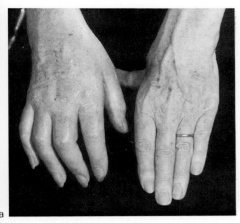
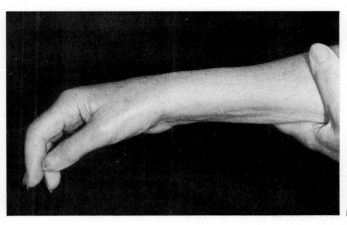

a                                                                                                                   b

**Fig. 4.13**   (a) Typical appearance of a hand suffering from reflex sympathetic dystrophy, demonstrating swelling, shiny skin and inability to fully extend the fingers, and (b) inability to flex the fingers.

Eventually the skin will change to a dry and shiny cyanosed colour and become cold. Porosis will show on X-ray and severe pain persists. Osteoporosis alone, however, is not sufficient evidence to make the diagnosis of a sympathetic dystrophy as it occurs from most severe hand injuries without any of the other signs and symptoms being present (Fig. 4.1).

Stiffness will inevitably result if the oedema and pain persist and the patient over-protects and does not use his hand (Fig. 4.13a & b). This disuse will also lead to muscle weakness.

Therapy can be beneficial in reducing pain in a proportion of cases. It may need to be combined with guanethidine blocks when the pain is particularly severe or if this does not succeed, a stellate ganglia block. A sympathectomy may eventually be necessary for those who do not respond to either form of treatment.

## Physiotherapy

Physiotherapy is invaluable both in the prevention of this disorder, and in its reversal during the very early stages. Later, if it has become established, it is a more difficult condition to treat successfully.

Prevention can be helped when immobilisation is necessary, by the correct positioning of the hand in the 'safe position' together with immediate active exercising of all available joints. Bombardment both peripherally and centrally by performing interesting functional activities will all help to retain normal sympathetic responses. Frequent checks should be made during the first few weeks following any injury or surgery that no dystrophy is developing. The patient must be warned to report immediately if the hand develops any of the recognised symptoms.

If a dystrophy does develop all means must be used to reverse the condition quickly. If the hand has had to be immobilised in a plaster of Paris cylinder it is advisable, if at all possible, that the cylinder is replaced with one made from a material that can be immersed in water. Contrast baths can then be given, which produce a sympathetic response to the changes of temperature. The cylinder should be replaced as early as possible by a splint which can be removed to allow free active exercising under supervision.

Elevation is imperative when oedema is present, as its reduction will assist in decreasing pain and improving mobility, besides preventing the development of fibrosis. The swollen hand and digit are made rigid by the excess fluid content, which can also be extremely painful. Ice dips or, if the patient prefers, the continuing use of contrast baths will help to reduce the swelling.

*Caution*. Interferential treatment has been found to increase the oedema that results from sympathetic dysfunction. PEMF and ultrasound are therefore preferable when treating pain and swelling if a dystrophy is suspected.

The patient must be encouraged to touch his affected hand or finger with his own normal, contralateral hand. Gentle active, but never passive, movements should be performed as fully as possible without causing the patient extreme pain. These treatments may be helped by the use of TNS to reduce the pain and discomfort. Electrodes should be positioned proximal to the affected part, over the appropriate nerve trunks. Dual output stimulators are therefore recommended.

When the patient can touch his hand for himself he must allow the therapist also to touch the painful area. He should then start moving his hand over different surfaces, using increasing pressure. Tapping movements onto first soft then harder surfaces, clapping hands, playing pat-a-cake, etc. should be commenced when possible.

If guanethidine blocks are introduced because of continuing pain, they should be followed immediately while the pain relief lasts, by similar treatment methods for reducing oedema and increasing activity. The blocks may need to be repeated several times if the effect is encouraging but short-lived. Therapists may have to urge patients to recover full range, especially if they have protected a painful hand for some time.

When the pain is under reasonable control the strength of activity should be increased. Accessory movements of the joints and gentle passive stretching should be given within the limits of pain, when there is residual stiffness. Stress should be laid increasingly on functional activities, and the occupational therapy department therefore plays an important role.

Severely painful hands can improve suddenly and dramatically, and in the majority of these cases motivation appears to be the important factor. The patient usually explains the improvement as stemming from his own determination to use his hand. For those that do not improve, a stellate ganglia block may then need to be performed.

## PERIPHERAL NERVE LESIONS

A correct diagnosis is most essential when a nerve lesion is involved so that the best management may be given. Some patients will need little more than assessment, advice and reappraisal. Others will need surgery and intensive physiotherapy for motor and sensory problems and for the complications arising from associated injuries.

## Causes

The main causes of nerve lesions are lacerations from glass and knives, the closed injuries of fractures and dislocations, ruptures as in brachial plexus lesions, and gunshot wound and blast injuries. Crush injuries, compression from too tight a plaster or bandage or a carpal tunnel syndrome, ischaemic injury and radiotherapy may all result in a nerve lesion. Drug abuse and over-indulgence in alcohol are occasional causes of nerve damage.

## Degeneration

Wallerian degeneration occurs following the division of a nerve. This is both to the proximal node of Ranvier and in the distal component of the nerve trunk. The debris from this degeneration is cleared away by macrophage activity and collagen is deposited gradually in the endoneurial tube. If re-innervation does not occur the muscle fibres also will be gradually replaced by fibrous tissue during the following 2–3 years.

## Regeneration

The axons sprout at the proximal stump of the nerve and, if no repair is attempted, they will form a neuroma. Regeneration takes place only if the nerve ends are in apposition.

Following a nerve repair these sprouting axons will attempt to regenerate into their original endoneurial tubes. This is rarely achieved correctly and some crossed re-innervation to both motor and sensory end-plates will inevitably result.

The average rate of peripheral nerve regeneration is about 1.0 to 1.5 mm a day, but is faster in children and usually slower in the elderly. It gradually slows when the site of the lesion is far from the skin and the muscles that need to be re-innervated. After 3 years the muscle fibres will have become irreversibly fibrosed, so that apart from some sensory recovery, very little functional ability will result.

## Effects of nerve injury

The effects of nerve damage are motor, sensory and autonomic.

*The motor effects* of a lower motor neurone lesion are loss of tone and reflexes and paralysis of muscles. Atrophy and deformities will develop, which if not treated will result in joint stiffness and contractures.

*The sensory effects* are loss of cutaneous and proprioceptive sensation. Some deep sensation will be saved if the tendons are intact. Deafferentation may lead to problems of pain. The area of sensory loss diminishes slightly when the adjacent normal nerves expand into the affected areas. Unless patients are warned, and constant reminders given, burns are liable to result.

*The autonomic effects* are changes in circulation and nutrition. The limb will take on the temperature of its surroundings and the affected skin area becomes pinkish-purple. Loss of sweating results and the skin is noticeably dry, first becoming scaly and later papery thin and shiny.

The poor nutrition induces deformity in the hair follicles, with a resulting effect on the hairs, the nails become ridged and the pulp of the finger tips reduces in size. Any cuts or blisters suffered due to loss of sensation may become trophic lesions and take many weeks to heal.

The area of skin affected is identical to that with sensory loss. It is therefore usually possible to identify the area of anaesthesia by observing the sympathetic changes.

## Types of nerve lesion

Neurapraxia, axonotmesis and neurotmesis are the main types of nerve injury.

*A neurapraxia* produces loss of conduction because of a block at site of injury. The distal component does not degenerate and when the cause of the lesion is removed there should be rapid recovery. There may be some sparing of crude sensation, and electromyographic (EMG) studies will show an absence of fibrillation potentials. Stimulation of the nerve trunk below the level of the lesion will elicit a normal muscle response, but this particular test must be delayed for 2 weeks in case any Wallerian degeneration occurs. This response differentiates a neurapraxia from an axonotmesis.

Physiotherapy for a neurapraxia should include assessment of joints, muscles and sensation and, if no EMG studies are available, the electrical stimulation of the nerve trunk distal to the site of the lesion. A neurapraxia should make an excellent recovery and the only treatment required should be to teach the patient the passive range of the joints involved, to instruct him on the necessary protection because of sensory loss, and to provide support to any flail joints. A description of the lesion and what to expect when recovery commences should be given and checks made frequently that the patient is maintaining his limb in good order. Spontaneous recovery should take place with return to completely normal function usually within 6 weeks, but occasionally it takes as long as 12 weeks.

*An axonotmesis* produces degeneration in the axons distal to the site of injury, but the sheath of the nerve is preserved. There is loss of conduction distal to the lesion and an EMG test will show both lack of volitional response and the presence of fibrillation potentials. Regeneration will commence when the cause of injury is removed, and usually a good recovery results.

Physiotherapy should include assessment of joints, muscles and sensation, and instruction on the effects of the lesion and protection necessary. When there is doubt as to the type of lesion in a closed injury and an EMG is not available the nerve trunk should be stimulated. If after 2 weeks this stimulation elicits no muscle response it suggests that degeneration has occurred. Any additional complications of fractures and dislocations also need physiotherapy treatment. Instruction should be given on care of the limb, passive movements and any signs of recovery that may be expected. Flail joints should be supported, preferably with lively splints. At the time of motor and sensory re-innervation an increase or some short bursts of treatment and re-education may be required for maximum results.

A mixed lesion of neurapraxia and axonotmesis can occur, some axons suffering degeneration but others being spared. An EMG will demonstrate fibrillation potentials of some muscle fibres, and yet conduction of others. A good recovery can be anticipated.

*A neurotmesis* involves the complete division of the nerve trunk and is usually found in conjunction with open injuries, fractures or traction lesions of the plexus. Loss of conduction occurs and EMG studies show similar results to those of an axonotmesis. Repair of a divided nerve is essential for regeneration, and the recovery time will again depend on the site of the lesion. The quality of recovery is frequently rather poor due to the inability of all axons to regenerate to their correct end-organs. Crossed re-innervation produces poor motor and sensory recovery with faulty localisation.

Assessment should be made of joints, muscles and sensation. There are likely to be more problems from associated injuries, such as lacerations, and incisions of skin and division of tendons and arteries. These may need intensive treatment in the early stages for oedema, pain and adherence of structures. Joints must be supported, passive movements taught and instructions given, both on protection of anaesthetic skin and on the progress expected. The intensity of treatment will need to be increased when recovery of muscles and sensation occurs, in order to maximise function.

N.B. If the lesion involves the plexus, any electrical tests performed by physiotherapists are likely to be of no significance. EMG tests are desirable to ensure an accurate diagnosis for peripheral nerve lesions. They are essential for plexus injuries.

### Repair

The best results of nerve repair follow primary nerve suture, as long as the wound is clean. Dirty wounds, which are liable to become infected, will cause poor nerve healing and regeneration, so that surgery should be delayed and a secondary repair performed. Frequently arteries will also have been divided and these should be repaired, if possible, and not ligated, in order to ensure an adequate circulation to the regenerating nerve.

With the advent of microsurgery precise techniques of suturing can now be performed. Choice of technique is usually between an epineurial or a fascicular repair. A gap in the nerve may necessitate the mobilisation of both proximal and distal ends to prevent a stretch being put on the repair. If the gap is larger than 2.5 mm a graft may be considered, but only if the bed for the graft is well vascularised. The result of grafting is usually less effective because the regenerating axons have two suture lines through which they must pass.

Immobilisation is usually for 3 weeks, as a stretch of the repaired ends is likely to jeopardise the re-

sults. Physiotherapy is then commenced, the therapist taking care not to place a passive stretch on the repair for a further 4 weeks.

Tendon transfers, either transferring the distal portion or the whole muscle together with its neurovascular supply, are techniques which may effectively restore function when nerve regeneration is unlikely. Occasionally a joint may need fusing in order to provide stability when the nerve does not recover and no transfers are possible.

### PHYSIOTHERAPY

Stages of treatment can be divided into early and recovery stages, although in practice they merge together.

### Early stage

Physiotherapy immediately following injury and surgery, which must include chest care, should concentrate on prevention of oedema, prevention of pain and the maintenance of joint mobility wherever possible. It is vital that the shoulder joint is exercised, especially in the elderly. A visual assessment can be made temporarily which includes active and passive movement as is applicable, but available joints and muscles should be measured as early as possible.

Most surgeons immobilise a sutured nerve for 3 weeks in order to allow healing and prevent any stretch on the approximated ends. To achieve some slackness of the nerve it may be necessary to position the joints in a loose-packed position, i.e. the wrist joint may be immobilised in flexion following median nerve suture. Extension is increased very gradually after 3–4 weeks.

Counselling during the first week or so should allow the patient to realise gradually the severity of his injury and likely length of time before full recovery. Emphasis must be laid on the support available and the eventual return of function so that he does not become too worried about the future.

After 3 weeks when the stitches are out and the immobilising splint has been removed, an assessment of motor, sensory and autonomic effects can be made. A sling may be necessary to reduce any oedema, and occasionally a splint is still needed to limit the stretch on the nerve ends for another few days. The splint, however, can usually be removed when the patient is assessed and treated in the physiotherapy department.

Joint range should now be measured and the total flexion and extension excursion of the fingers recorded. The effect that the scar has on tendon function should be observed carefully in case any adhesions prevent full flexion, full extension or possibly both. A laceration that divides a nerve will frequently have divided muscle, tendons and other tissues. The divided structures lie in layers directly one above the other and after surgery they may have become adherent, skin to tendons, and tendons to each other, and to the deeper structures such as capsules and ligaments. This problem can limit movement considerably, and will need a great intensity of treatment during early rehabilitation.

Pain, when still present after 2–3 weeks, needs urgent treatment as it is more difficult to cure when it has become long standing. Spontaneous firing of discharges may occur at the proximal stump of the nerve and there can be no afferent inhibition from the divided section. In partial and recovering peripheral nerve lesions painful paraesthesia and causalgia may result together, in severe cases, with hyperpathia. If neuromata form at the proximal stump there will also be an increase of these painful spontaneous discharges in the afferents.

TNS, if applied early after injury, is effective in a large portion of cases. The electrodes must be positioned on an area where sensation is still present. Pain is frequently experienced in the anaesthetic areas and they should therefore be placed proximal to the site of the lesion, over the nerve trunk. Several attempts may have to be made on consecutive days to find the most effective positions for the electrodes. The duration of treatment should be at least 2 hours and preferably more, to be beneficial but TNS can be used safely for as long as the patient desires. If pain is persistent however guanethidine blocks may be needed, combined with vigorous therapy, to reduce the pain to an acceptable level. Distraction, by involvement in leisure interests and games etc., when combined with more formal treatment is one of the best ways of coping, as higher centre inhibition is produced. The patient must assess his pain daily for himself on the 10 centimetre scale, recording

the duration of any relief from the previous day's treatment in order to achieve the optimum result.

Scars and their surrounding areas will need softening. Massage, PEMF and U/S are all useful. Webs should not be forgotten, as they quickly contract and will need regular stretching.

If movement is limited by adhesions it is possible that joints may stiffen also. Joint mobility must therefore be maintained; at the same time the therapist should ensure that the suture is not jeopardised by stretch. Tension can be slackened by flexing both wrist and MCP joints, thereby allowing the IP joints to extend automatically. Similarly, by flexing both the wrist and IP joints the MCP joints will also extend easily. The presence of adhesions should not usually be sufficient excuse for the development of joint stiffness.

Adhesions may be stretched actively, i.e. by the patient himself, usually after 3–4 weeks, as long as the stretch applied is very gentle. No passive stretch should be given to sutured structures at this stage. Active movements should gradually increase in power, with resistance added at 5–6 weeks. A passive stretch may be safely given at 8 weeks.

Power of the proximal muscles must be remembered. If the muscles of the hand are paralysed the strength of the shoulder girdle, shoulder and elbow will inevitably be reduced. Similarly the muscles that are antagonistic to those affected by the lesion will weaken unless specific exercise is given. The use of lively splints helps to maintain function of these antagonists.

Joints without active control should be supported both to prevent a prolonged stretch of ligaments and capsule, which can be very painful, and to prevent adaptive shortening of the unopposed muscles: for example, in a radial nerve injury the wrist should be supported in a cock-up splint. Similarly a recovering nerve, especially if divided and sutured, should not be left on a stretch as this will reduce recovery. Muscles will become inhibited if subjected to prolonged stretch. The normal position of rest for wrist, fingers and thumb is suitable when support is necessary whilst awaiting nerve regeneration.

Lively splints form a useful adjunct during the management of nerve lesions. Their main applications are:

1. To provide support for joints and soft tissues,

thereby preventing deformities and contractures.

2. To improve function by:
   a. Placing the hand in a functional position, e.g. wrist cock-up splint.
   b. Utilising alternative muscle action, e.g. in a combined median and ulnar nerve lesion, if the MCP joints are held in very slight flexion, EDC is able to extend the IP joints. This activity also prevents the claw deformity.
   c. Directly replacing muscle function, e.g. a spider splint extends the MCP joints in a radial nerve lesion.
   d. Exercising antagonist activity.

If either lively or static splints are used the patient must be instructed to remove the splint regularly and mobilise the hand through the full passive range. The author has treated a patient to whom this instruction was not given following a radial nerve lesion. His hand had become totally extended with joints rigid and muscles contracted. It took several months of intensive treatment to rectify the condition.

Counselling is essential at this stage, with instructions given to the patient so that he understands the purpose of normal nerve supply, the effects of its damage, the recovery expected, and the care necessary whilst waiting for nerve regeneration. Motor and sensory effects should be identified and compared with the contralateral limb. It is important that the patient understands that increased wasting will occur and that there will be an inevitable time lapse before re-innervation commences. Any occupational or social problems should be discovered quickly so that action can be taken.

### Recovery stage

Assessments to discover any return of muscle activity and sensation should be increased when re-innervation is anticipated. An estimation of this event can be made by measuring the distance of injury from area to be re-innervated and calculating the likely time for recovery. A millimetre a day is the average rate of regeneration. The Tinel test usually helps to indicate both site of injury and point of regeneration.

Activity should first be tested in those muscles expected to be normal, followed by those expected to be affected by the lesion and all should be graded on the 0–5 scale. Trick movements and anomalies should be anticipated. Sensation should be charted using different colour codes for normal, anaesthetic and altered sensation.

Increased treatment should be given when muscle flickers are discovered. Sometimes muscles that show no activity at the time of assessment will start to contract if bombarded for several days with physiological input. The nerves have a high threshold following regeneration, which necessitates this increased facilitation. PNF techniques of treatment are therefore very appropriate. Computerised games with EMG bio-feedback, using surface electrodes, are usually most helpful to the patient. Repeated sessions of these techniques for maximising muscle function will be necessary for up to three years, depending on the distance of the lesion from the muscles needing re-innervation. After 3 years the muscle recovery is likely to be minimal, and surgery may be the only means by which function can be restored (see p. 167).

During this stage of recovery, observation should be made for any deterioration in the deformities. In a high level lesion of the median and ulnar nerves clawing will increase when the long muscles to the fingers recover. It is urgent that adequate passive movement and stretching is given, and taught to the patient, in order to prevent contractures.

Lively or static splinting may still be needed, but should be discarded when not essential. Sometimes muscles that have recently recovered may tire by the end of the day, at which time the splint can still be useful. At work it may be necessary to stabilise or support a part until muscle strength improves.

Sensory return needs to be monitored by therapists at regular intervals following a median nerve lesion in order to commence re-education as early as possible and thus maximise function. Cotton wool or even the light touch of a finger tip is an appropriate means, the therapist taking great care not to produce a joint movement. Hyperaesthesia is experienced in the palm first, gradually reaching the finger tips, and thus giving some protective sensation. The pins and needles are uncomfortable for the patient but he should be told that it is an indication of nerve recovery and should soon change to more normal sensation. The hyperaesthesia is due to immaturity of the myelin. In most people this deficiency is eventually corrected, but with the more elderly it sometimes remains a big problem. TNS can be beneficial by lessening the pins and needles sensation, but will probably need to be used daily. These patients should, ideally, have their own stimulator.

Surgeons also need an assessment of the quality of their nerve repairs by the measurement of sensory regeneration. Tests, with the therapists using different diameter monofilaments or a Von Frey hair, are both subjective and time consuming, and do not assess sensory function. The development of a simple EMG sensory conduction test and the measurement of skin resistance by sweat meter may provide a rapid and more accurate answer in the future.

The static 2 point discrimination test has been found to bear very little relationship to function (Wynn Parry & Salter 1976). Static touch receptors, which are slow adapting, are the last to regenerate after nerve repair and in fact frequently do not regenerate at all, probably due to lack of sufficient axoplasm (Wynn Parry 1984). The rapid adapting mechanoreceptors, that are stimulated by a moving touch, are however likely to recover. 2 point discrimination, if included, should therefore be measured by a moving touch (Dellon 1984). Similarly localisation should be tested with a moving finger touch and the results charted.

Sensory re-education should commence when there is normal sensation in the palm, but some residual hyperaesthesia in the finger tips. It should start with different shapes of wood and large objects, thus mainly utilising proprioception for recognition. When the cutaneous sensation of the finger tips becomes normal the size of the objects should be decreased and different textures and materials introduced (p. 100). Improved stereognostic ability is due to the flow of more normal sensory discharges from the recovered tactile receptors. Less information is gained from the proprioceptors when handling small objects and different textures, and the ability to recognise these is therefore dependent on cutaneous recovery. It is essential that both these aspects of sensory ability are considered during re-education. Training must also be included to correct any faulty localisation in the median distribution following nerve repair.

Leprosy patients frequently suffer incurable cutaneous anaesthesia, but some proprioception may remain. This is gained from any muscles, tendons and joints that may still have a normal nerve supply, and should therefore be utilised for stereognosis training. Emphasis should be particularly on discriminating between different shapes, sizes and weights of objects. By watching and then repeating the action with his eyes closed the patient should be able to gain a more efficient idea of what his hand is doing, and this should help him to protect himself when performing activities that could be damaging to his anaesthetic skin.

## SPECIFIC NERVE LESIONS

The lesions described include those of radial, median and ulnar, and the combined median and ulnar nerve lesions, with a mention of brachial plexus lesions as these affect the hand in a proportion of cases.

### Radial nerve lesions

The radial nerve supplies those muscles which extend and stabilise both elbow, wrist and fingers. Acting as fixators they position the wrist in sufficient extension so that the finger flexors can contract strongly. Active extension movements are necessary for grasp, first to stretch the fingers round the object and later to release it. The radial nerve is responsible for this extension control.

The nerve is most frequently damaged by fractures of the shaft of the humerus, involving it in its spiral groove. It can also be affected by pressure in the axilla. The muscles involved are supinator, brachio-radialis, extensor carpi ulnaris, extensor carpi radialis longus and brevis, extensor digitorum communis, extensors indicis and digiti minimi, extensors pollicis longus and brevis and abductor pollicis longus. Lesions have to be close to the axilla to affect the triceps.

The result is a wrist drop combined with loss of MCP joint extension of the fingers and of extension and abduction of the thumb (Fig. 4.14a). Some supination will be preserved because of biceps action.

*The trick movements* include extension of the IP joints of the fingers by the intrinsic muscles when the MCP joints are supported and stabilised in extension by the examiner. A dipping action of the

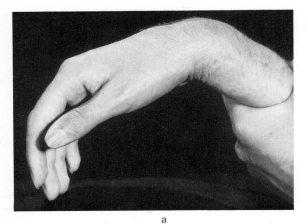

a

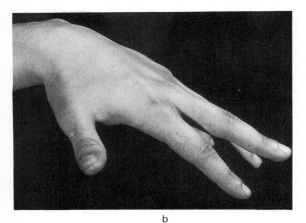

b

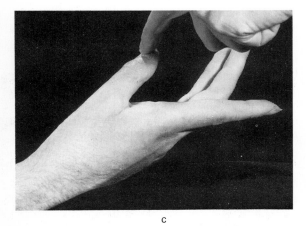

c

**Fig. 4.14** A radial nerve lesion causes: (a) The drop-wrist deformity; (b) Dipping of the wrist into full flexion to produce MCP and IP joint extension by the tenodesis action; (c) Extension of the IP joint of the thumb by a contraction of abductor pollicis brevis with its slip insertion into the dorsal expansion.

whole hand occurs when the patient is asked to extend his fingers, without any support being given. This enables him to extend both MCP and IP joints by tenodesis action (Fig. 4.14b). The wrist is actively flexed downwards and held in full flexion, which has a tautening effect on the long extensors of the fingers, and a passive extension of MCP and IP joints therefore occurs. Conversely, some wrist extension may sometimes be produced, again by a tenodesis action, as the result of full and strong finger flexion. The tautening effect on the finger extensors will in this instance pull the wrist back into slight extension. Extension of the IP joint of the thumb can be produced by APB, with its normal median nerve supply, because of its slip insertion into the dorsal expansion of the thumb. At the same time it pulls the thumb into abduction and rotation (Fig. 4.14c). If held beside the index finger a small degree of extension of the IP joint may still be possible, and it is therefore advisable to leave the thumb free when testing EPL and look for a correct movement, a contraction of the tendon and the absence of abduction. These trick movements may not be immediately apparent if the hand and forearm are in a plaster of Paris which extends slightly beyond the MCP joints of fingers and thumb.

Injury at the level of the forearm can cause damage to the posterior interosseous nerve (see p. 145) and to the sensory nerve also, where it passes superficially over the shaft of the radius at the junction of mid and lower thirds, making it rather vulnerable. The sensory distribution is variable: it may supply the major part of the skin of the dorsum of the hand (radial side), or only a small area at the base of the thumb (p. 13). Occasionally there is no sensory distribution at all from the radial nerve.

Typical posture of the patient presenting with a radial nerve lesion is a hand held in supination, thus eliminating the wrist drop which can, after some weeks, become very uncomfortable due to the stretch on the ligaments and capsule. The effect on the function of the hand is mainly from the loss of wrist extension combined with the difficulty of grasp and release of large objects because the fingers cannot be extended.

*Physiotherapy* is concerned with maintaining mobility of joints and muscles at first, and re-education later.

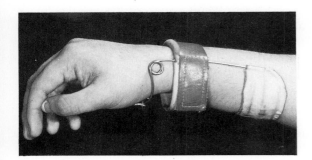

**Fig. 4.15** A lively cock-up splint for preventing the wrist drop.

A simple cock-up splint is essential to support the wrist after a radial nerve lesion and can be either static or lively (Fig. 4.15). The complicated form of splint which suspends the fingers and thumb in extension tends to hinder function, and flatten the arches. It is cosmetically undesirable and makes dressing extremely difficult. In most circumstances it should not be used. The semi-flexed posture of the fingers, with the thumb slightly abducted and rotated, is a natural resting position for the hand, but the wrist must always be supported in some extension.

Function can frequently be improved by the addition of a spider splint for the fingers, worn in conjunction with either a static or lively cock-up splint for the wrist. The spider splint allows the fingers to flex fully (Fig. 4.16a) and finger extension is provided by the spring action of the splint when the finger flexors relax (Fig. 4.16b). The

amount of extension available is usually enough to allow grasp round the largest sized objects and, as an additional attraction, the splint is easily pocketed when not needed. The lively cock-up splint is not visible when worn under a sleeve, so that this combination of splints is very acceptable to most patients.

In a *lesion of the posterior interosseous nerve*, when activity of both brachioradialis and extensor carpi radialis longus is preserved, wrist extension remains, albeit with a bias of radial deviation due to lack of activity in extensor carpi ulnaris. The hand can function quite efficiently if some metacarpophalangeal joint extension is provided by a spider splint.

*During muscle re-innervation* brachioradialis is usually first to recover followed by extensor carpi radialis longus and brevis, and then the supinator. Recovery of extensor carpi ulnaris corrects the bias of radial deviation and is followed usually by recovery of finger extension. The MCP joints of the index and little fingers are frequently found to extend initially through a greater range than the other fingers. This is because of the additional contraction of extensor indicis, or extensor digiti minimi, with extensor digitorum. The thumb is usually the last to recover its muscle power, and the earliest sign of recovery in EPL is usually the decrease of palmar abduction when attempting to extend the terminal joint.

Splintage should be reduced when the strength improves and the patient can manage without support. This may be suitable for only part of the

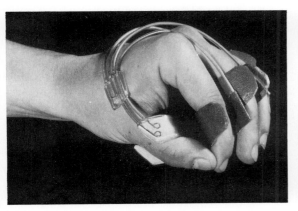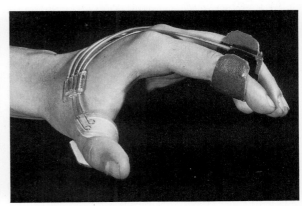

**Fig. 4.16** (a) The spider splint allows full active flexion. (b) Extension, gained on relaxation of the flexors, enables grasp and release of objects. The splint is easily pocketed.

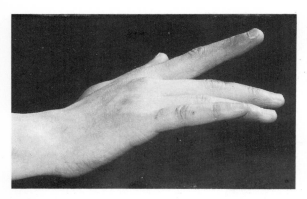

**Fig. 4.17** Recovery of finger extension after a radial nerve lesion is often seen first in index and little fingers because of the additional power provided by extensors indicis and minimus.

day but a delay in removing the splint may otherwise slow progress.

If the injury to the radial nerve is at a high level there will be a considerable time lapse before muscle re-innervation occurs. If this is likely to be a very long time and there is some doubt over the effectiveness of recovery, tendon transfer procedures may be performed as a suitable means for returning some function to the arm. If the extensor muscles recover later there is no real disadvantage to the patient.

*Residual problems* following a radial nerve lesion are mainly from lack of re-innervation of the extensor muscles. There is usually a delay of several months between injury and recovery, so that corrective procedures should be considered when re-innervation is expected but does not actually happen. Wrist extension, and thumb and finger extension combined with abduction, are the most essential functions to restore. Sensory loss in the radial distribution only is not a very great problem to the patient.

Pronator teres, flexor carpi ulnaris and palmaris longus are commonly used as donors for tendon transfer procedures. They are sutured into extensor carpi radialis brevis, extensor digitorum communis and extensor pollicis longus, and abductor pollicis longus respectively. A splint provides support for three weeks in order to prevent too much stretch to the donor muscles. Very gentle exercise may, with the surgeon's agreement, be commenced one week after surgery, but this is frequently delayed

for 3 weeks. Re-education of the muscles to an altered role is not usually difficult (see p. 167) and most results are excellent. Lack of extension as the result of a brachial plexus lesion may be more difficult to restore, however.

## Median nerve lesions

Delicate and skilled function of the hand is achieved by the combination of an excellent motor and sensory supply, which is largely gained from the median nerve distribution. Skin receptors are particularly dense in the skin on the ulnar side of the thumb and the radial side of the index finger, and these areas are highly represented on the sensory cortex. Activities such as tying up shoe-laces, doing up buttons, writing, and painting, are those that suffer most in an injury to the median nerve.

The nerve is especially vulnerable at the wrist where it lies superficial only to skin and the palmaris longus tendon. It is most commonly injured by lacerations at this site together usually with one or more tendons. It can also be affected by compression in the carpal tunnel.

With a lesion at wrist level the muscles affected are abductor pollicis brevis, opponens pollicis, the superficial head of flexor pollicis brevis, and the lateral (radial) two lumbricals. The thenar muscles become increasingly wasted so that the flat or monkey hand deformity develops, with the thumb lying lateral instead of anterior to the index finger (Fig. 4.18a). This is caused by the unopposed actions of extensor pollicis longus and adductor pollicis. There may also be a very slight claw deformity of the index and middle fingers due to inactivity of the two lumbricals, but the normal action of the interossei to these two fingers prevents this from becoming pronounced.

The volar surfaces of the thumb, index, middle and radial side of the ring finger will be anaesthetic, together with the dorsal surfaces of the same digits from the level of the proximal interphalangeal joints to the tips of the digits. Autonomic changes, including loss of sweating, change of colour and change of skin texture, will be observed in the same distribution (Fig. 4.18a). Atrophy of the thumb web will quickly develop if not well mobilised.

Flexion of the thumb is preserved but during attempted opposition FPB can only flex the thumb

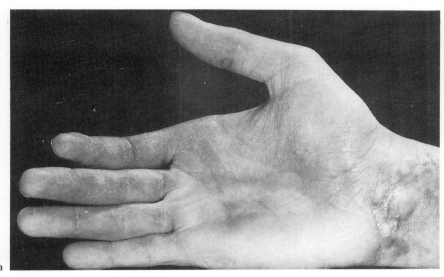
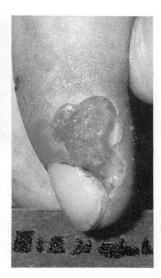

a                                                                                      b

**Fig. 4.18**  (a) A lesion of the median nerve clearly shows the cutaneous distribution. (b) A patient who burnt his finger on a lighted cigarette.

towards the base of the little finger while remaining in contact with the palm (Fig. 4.19a) as the rotation of the metacarpal and the normally powerful thrust of the thenar eminence muscles are both lost. This is because of the paralysis of the thenar muscles which normally position the thumb in some abduction. An attempt to make an 'O' with

index finger and thumb usually results in a very flat 'D' being formed (Fig. 4.19c).

The trick movement of palmar abduction may occasionally be possible due to a combined or alternating contraction of abductor pollicis longus, with its radial nerve supply, and the deep head of flexor pollicis brevis, with an ulnar nerve supply

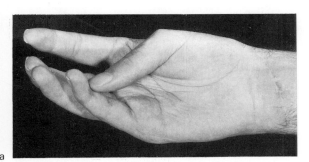

a

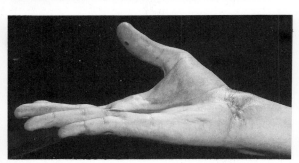

b

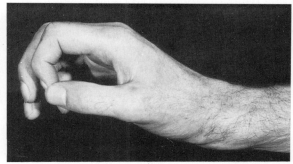

c

**Fig. 4.19**  In median nerve lesions: (a) Attempted opposition involving flexion and rotation at the carpometacarpal joint is replaced by increased flexion at the metacarpophalangeal joint. The little finger flexes increasingly towards the tip of thumb. (b) Trick palmar abduction of the thumb produced by a combined contraction of the deep head of flexor pollicis brevis·and abductor pollicis longus. (c) The very flat 'D' produced when attempting to form an 'O'.

(Fig. 4.19b). It is, however, a rather weak and unstable movement.

A lesion at the level of the wrist should show signs of returning muscle activity at approximately 90 days after suture. Abductor pollicis brevis is the muscle which usually contracts first. An improvement in the position in which the thumb lies is often the first sign of recovery, before a flicker of movement can be observed. Active movement will follow but it usually takes some weeks or months, if at all, before the thumb can perform sufficiently well to touch the little finger in a normal and strong movement pattern.

Lesions of the median nerve at the level of or above the elbow can be caused by lacerations, ischaemia, fractures and traction of the roots. The pre-mentioned muscles of the hand are involved and also the forearm and finger flexors. These include pronator teres, flexor carpi radialis, palmaris longus (if present) and flexor digitorum superficialis. The anterior interosseous branch, which is given off just below the elbow, and which occasionally is damaged in isolation, supplies flexor digitorum profundus (FDP) to either both index and middle fingers or to index alone, flexor pollicis longus and pronator quadratus.

The deformity produced by a median nerve lesion at high level is that of the pointing finger (Fig. 4.20a) when the nerve supplies FDP to only the index, or the position of benediction if it supplies FDP to both index and middle fingers. Contraction of FDP to the other two (or three) fingers is preserved through the supply from the ulnar nerve. Sensory and autonomic distribution is the same as in a lesion at the wrist. Adaptations or lively splints may be used for improving function of an anterior interosseous nerve lesion (Fig. 4.20).

Early signs of recovery at high level include a slight return of pronation and wrist flexion. A contraction of flexor carpi radialis can be felt over the tendon at the wrist. Flexion of the fingers returns before flexion of the thumb, and the last of the forearm muscles to recover is pronator quadratus. If the level of a median nerve lesion is at the elbow there will inevitably be a long delay before recovery can occur in both muscles and sensation of the hand.

*Physiotherapy* is important early for maintaining the passive range of joints, the suppleness of the

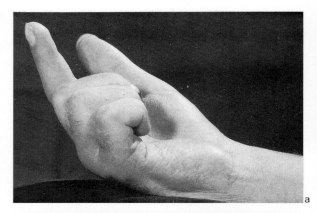

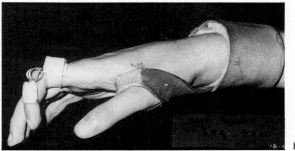

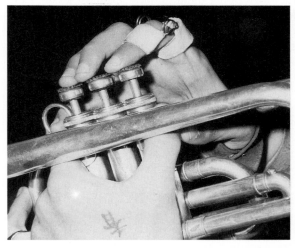

**Fig. 4.20** (a) The pointing finger of the high median nerve lesion. (b & c) Lively splints may be used to improve function.

webs and the prevention of gross thenar eminence deformity. Provision of a lively splint made of Neoprene, which pulls the thumb into some abduction and opposition, will help to prevent an excessive deformity (Fig. 4.20b). It also assists function as the finger tips can be flexed towards the suitably positioned thumb. Repeated warnings must be given regarding the sensory loss (Fig. 4.18b).

It is more difficult to assist function if the lesion is at a high level, when it involves the finger and wrist flexors. Gross deformity of the thenar eminence must be prevented, however, by the use of the above mentioned splint.

If the webs, particularly of the thumb, have become contracted, intensive treatment must be given. Passive stretching and the use of wedges, preferably of Polyform, should improve the degree of passive abduction. If the circulation is so poor that Polyform is not suitable, Plastazote can be used instead. It may be necessary to treat the web to increase both palmar and radial abduction, and if so, separate splints will be needed to maintain each position. Polyform is most suited for this purpose as it moulds perfectly round the digits, thus holding the required position exactly.

The wrist and finger flexors must be re-educated immediately a flicker of movement is discovered, and gradually strengthened during the following weeks. The extensors may also be found to be weak due to complete lack of hand function, and therefore will need strengthening.

Facilitation techniques are extremely important when re-educating thumb movements. The thenar muscles should be exercised in outer range at first as recovering muscles are unable to contract through full range in the early stages. Excursion should gradually increase as strength returns.

Sensory re-education should commence immediately there is some hyperaesthesia in the tips of the thumb, index and middle fingers and a more normal sensation in the palm. The normal area of skin supplied by the ulnar nerve must be covered by Tubigrip or finger stalls as otherwise the patient will only use this part of his hand. A blindfold or mask will ensure that the patient cannot see what he is feeling.

Although the return of cutaneous sensation is necessary for stereognosis a great deal of the gnostic ability is from proprioception. If a lesion of a median nerve is in conjunction with that of the radial nerve and particularly when at high level, there will be an enormous disability. Proprioception from joint receptors and tendons will be greatly reduced and patients frequently complain of dropping objects. In lesions of the median nerve alone, however, use can be made of the residual proprioceptive feedback available from the tendons, muscles and joints with a normal nerve supply. Large objects that are simple to manipulate are fairly easily recognised during early sensory recovery. Small objects and materials are recognised much later, because the proprioceptive in-put when handling these items is imperceptible. Stereognosis is then dependent almost entirely on feedback from the cutaneous receptors. Any incorrect localisation will also need retraining in order to improve stereognostic function.

Sensation cannot be divorced from movement, so that functional activities will help to improve stereognosis, and conversely practical sensory training will improve co-ordination of movement. These facts should be utilised in all treatments, whether concentrating on muscle activity or on sensory re-education.

*Residual problems* of a median nerve lesion may include permanent lack of hypothenar muscle re-innervation. The resulting loss of normal thumb movement especially palmar abduction and opposition may seriously handicap some patients whilst others may manage without too much difficulty. An opponens transfer can restore function to the thumb but only if sufficient sensation is present to ensure that an operative procedure will be worthwhile. An alternative to surgery is to make permanent use of a median lively splint, which provides some degree of opposition. This splint is described on p. 114.

Failure of sensory recovery when the skin of thumb, index and middle fingers remains anaesthetic, is an extremely severe disability. At time of injury, when the gap in the nerve is too great for local mobilisation, a section of sural nerve may be used for a graft. Occasionally the ulnar or radial nerve may be sacrificed to graft into the distal portion of the ulnar, but this is an extreme decision to make. Finally, if sensory recovery does not occur, but motor function is good, some neurovascular skin island transfers may be performed using skin with ulnar nerve supply. This is taken usually from the ring finger and transposed complete with neurovascular bundles to thumb and index tips. Unfortunately, it has the effect of transferring the donor localisation also. Unless intensive sensory re-education is given to correct this localisation problem the patient is unlikely to use his hand. He will continue to feel that he is using his ring finger and not his index finger and thumb.

Permanent hyperaesthesia is a problem that can often be relieved by the use of TNS. If pain, however, remains intense, and is not helped by either TNS or guanethidine blocks, the patient may need to attend a pain clinic for alternative treatment to be considered.

## Ulnar nerve lesions

Power and stability of the hand, together with co-ordination, are gained to a great extent from the ulnar nerve distribution. Activities such as typing and piano playing are severely affected by an ulnar nerve lesion due to the loss of lateral movements of the fingers together with decreased sensory feedback. Inability to elevate the head of the 5th metacarpal and oppose the little finger towards the thumb impairs power grip considerably and articles slide through the hand. Loss of stability of the index finger and thumb severely reduces all types of pinch grip and activities such as cutting meat, when the index finger normally steadies and directs the shaft of the knife. The support normally provided for the hand by resting on the little finger is reduced because abductor digiti minimi is paralysed and the skin is anaesthetic. If patients complain of difficulty in maintaining grasp of a hammer or a racquet it may be due not only to weakened muscles but also to poor proprioception.

The ulnar nerve is most frequently damaged by lacerations at the wrist, often by putting the hand through a window, when tendons and the ulnar artery also are liable to be severed. When the nerve and tendons are sutured it is essential that the artery is repaired and not ligated, as an adequate circulation is necessary to ensure good regeneration of the nerve.

A lesion at wrist level affects abductor digiti minimi, flexor and opponens digiti minimi, adductor pollicis, all the interossei, and the lumbricals to ring and little fingers. The volar surfaces of the little and the adjacent half of the ring finger will become anaesthetic but sensation on the dorsal aspect, except for the tips of these fingers, will be spared (Fig. 2.13). This is because the dorsal cutaneous branch of the ulnar nerve is given off in the lower third of the forearm, and therefore is usually proximal to the wrist laceration.

Wasting results in the hypothenar eminence and in the interosseous spaces, and is particularly noticeable in the thumb web. The claw hand deformity gradually develops with the diminishing tone of the paralysed muscles, and the arches flatten (Fig. 4.21a & b). The combined action of the long extensors and the long flexors of the fingers produce extension of the MCP joints and flexion of the IP joints of ring and little fingers. As the muscles of these two fingers are unopposed, the claw or intrinsic minus deformity develops. It is the interossei that normally provide flexion of the MCP and extension of the IP joints. A patient with an ulnar nerve lesion can usually hold his index and middle fingers in this position by using his median supplied lumbricals (Fig. 4.21c). If their power is tested, however, by giving even the slightest resistance, the fingers will collapse. This helps to endorse the fact that it is the interossei and not the lumbricals which produce this normally powerful intrinsic movement. When asked to extend the hand and then make a fist it will be seen that the ring and little fingers move in a clawing fashion. Normally in flexion and extension movements, the MCP joints flex at the same time as the IP joints, and conversely all joints extend together. This helps the fingers to reach around an object as the tips are held away from the palm by the lumbrical action. In an ulnar nerve lesion the IP joints of ring and little fingers flex first, followed by the MCP joints in a rolling movement, which is termed 'rolling flexion'. During extension the MCP joints of ring and little fingers extend first and any attempt to extend the IP joints will result in the claw deformity. The normal action of the median supplied lumbricals will prevent this clawing effect on the index and middle fingers. With the paralysis of the hypothenar muscles it becomes impossible to raise the head of the fifth metacarpal and to oppose the little finger towards the thumb (Fig. 4.21d).

*The trick movements* seen in an ulnar nerve lesion include a small amount of abduction and adduction of the fingers, which is possible when performing as a group. Abduction occurs in conjunction with finger extension and is produced by extensor digitorum. Adduction, together with some finger flexion, is provided by flexor digitorum profundus and superficialis. Both abduction and adduction are brought about because of the angles

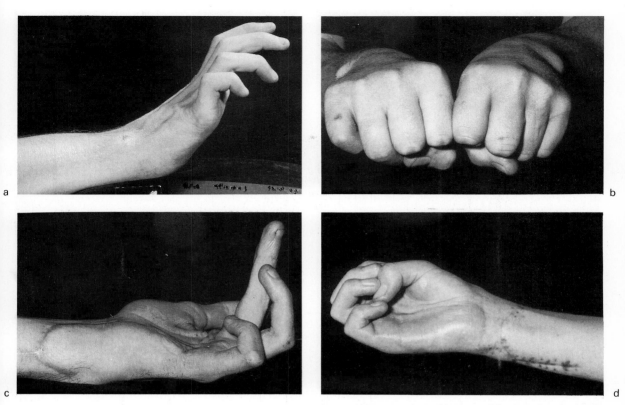

**Fig. 4.21** The classical ulnar nerve lesion: (a) showing the claw hand deformity, with (b) flattening of the transverse arches, (c) the inability to flex the MCP joints and extend the IP joints of ring and little fingers, (d) the inability to raise the head of the fifth metacarpal in order to oppose the little finger towards the thumb.

formed by the tendons as they lie over the MCP joints. When the muscles contract, pulling the tendons straight, a lateral movement is produced at all the MCP joints except that of the middle finger. The muscles should therefore be tested not only in a group action but each finger individually. With the palm resting on the table the patient is asked to extend and then abduct and adduct each finger in turn. In the normal hand it is simple to perform a full lateral movement: with an ulnar nerve lesion it is impossible. The index finger may produce just a few degrees of movement, however, by contracting first extensor indicis followed by extensor digitorum to the index finger, when contractions of these tendons can be seen over the dorsum of the MCP joint, flicking from one to the other and back again (Fig. 4.22a & b).

Any attempt to abduct and adduct the middle finger individually will produce a totally different type of trick movement. The patient will probably be able to move the tip of his middle finger first nearer the index and then nearer the ring finger, not by a normal movement but from a lateral shift of the whole palm. When observed carefully it will be seen that the joints that actually move are both the wrist and the MCP joints of the other three fingers. In fact no movement takes place at all at the required joint, i.e. the MCP joint of the middle finger. The same trick movement will be seen with the ring finger. In the little finger, however, the presence of two extensor tendons may enable a lateral movement to be performed similar to that seen in the index finger.

A further trick movement is seen when the patient is asked to adduct his thumb. A strong contraction at the same time of both flexor pollicis longus and extensor pollicis longus will adduct the thumb (Fig. 4.22c). This again is because of the angle of

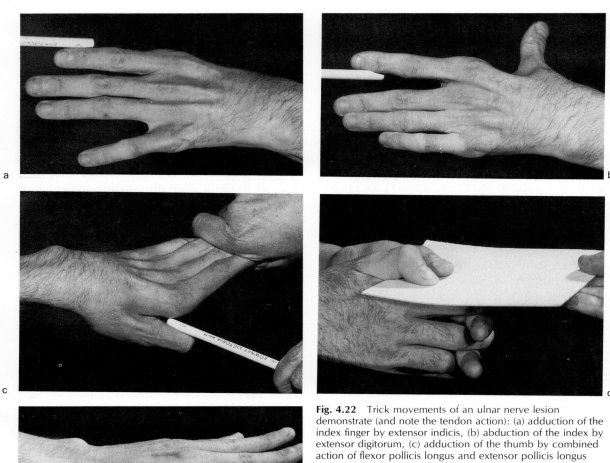

a

b

c

d

e

**Fig. 4.22** Trick movements of an ulnar nerve lesion demonstrate (and note the tendon action): (a) adduction of the index finger by extensor indicis, (b) abduction of the index by extensor digitorum, (c) adduction of the thumb by combined action of flexor pollicis longus and extensor pollicis longus (note the excessive wasting of the interosseous spaces) and also the activity of EPL. (d) Froment's sign demonstrates excessive IP joint flexion of the thumb in order to pinch onto a card. This patient's flexion deformities necessitated the linking of his fingers. (e) Recovery in the same patient, 5 months later, when muscle bulk has returned, the MCP joints are no longer hyper-extended and the thumb adduction has resumed a normal pattern.

pull of the tendons. Sometimes the patient performs this movement with the thumb extended and sometimes with it flexed. The extensor tendon jumps over the MCP joint as the thumb adducts, resulting in a jerky movement. If pinch grip is tested by using a stiff card while the palms are placed together, normal thumb adduction is replaced by pronounced IP joint flexion (Fig. 4.22d). This is known as Froment's sign. Tip grip is also reduced considerably because of the paralysis of both the adductor pollicis and the 1st dorsal interosseous muscle. It can be illustrated when an attempt is

made to form an 'O' between index and thumb when the index finger is unable to stabilise itself without fully flexing the PIP joint. This is different from the median nerve lesion, where it is the thumb that is unable to abduct and rotate sufficiently to form the 'O'.

A laceration of the palm may divide the deep branch of the ulnar nerve after it has given off its supply to abductor digiti minimi and the other hypothenar muscles. The superficial branch supplying the digital nerves may also be involved. Very careful motor and sensory assessments should be performed as early as possible after this type of injury as nerve damage may easily be overlooked. Surgery, if it is needed to repair the nerve branches, should ideally be performed before too much fibrosis can occur. Compression or constant trauma can also cause damage to both deep and superficial branches of the nerve. The cause should be removed to allow recovery to take place.

Lesions of the nerve around or above the level of the elbow will affect flexor carpi ulnaris and flexor digitorum profundus to the ring and little fingers and also those muscles of the hand already discussed. Sensation will be lost over both dorsal and volar surfaces on the medial side of the hand and fingers.

Initially the claw deformity of the fingers is not so pronounced in a high level ulnar nerve injury as in a lesion at the wrist, due to the paralysis of flexor digitorum profundus (FDP). At the stage when FDP recovers, however, the deformity may worsen.

Recovery in the small muscles of the hand is first indicated at approximately 80 days after injury at the wrist, when the little finger starts to drift into increasing abduction. This is caused by returning activity of abductor digiti minimi (ADM) which is unopposed by the still paralysed interossei. A contraction in ADM should soon be sufficient to be palpated. Recovery of the interossei and lumbricals is often rather poor, and rarely do individual abduction and adduction of the fingers fully return. The claw deformity gradually decreases, however, and a more normal flexion and extension pattern of the fingers can be observed. If the physiotherapist places the ring and little fingers with MCP joints flexed and IP joints extended the patient may be able to hold them in position for a second or two before the fingers collapse. Adduction of the thumb will take on a more normal pattern of movement, and lose its jerky trick action (Fig. 4.22e).

*Physiotherapy* is concerned in the early stages with maintaining mobility of joints and soft tissues. It is important that the claw deformity is stretched out regularly, that the arches are maintained passively and the webs stretched. A lively splint should be worn that will prevent hyperextension of MCP joints of the ring and little fingers (Wynn Parry 1981). If these joints are stabilised in very slight flexion the extensor digitorum is able to pull through and extend the interphalangeal joints. The patient can thus correct his own claw deformity by means of the splint (Fig. 4.23a) but he should not be expected to wear one that is clumsy (Fig. 4.23b).

As much time as is suitable should be spent in re-educating the affected muscles when recovery is seen. Facilitation techniques help to maximise function in these small muscles which may, until sensory feedback is applied, appear to be inactive. Approximation given through the MCP joints, when positioning them in some flexion, and through the IP joints, when placing them in extension, makes the patient more aware of the position he is trying to hold. Lateral movements of the fingers and opposition of the little finger towards the thumb should be facilitated by use of stretch. At first the muscles can only contract in their outer range; the range and power will improve slowly over the following weeks. Short bursts of intensive treatment repeated fairly frequently have been found

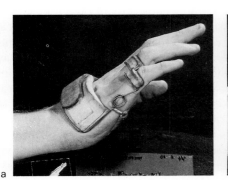
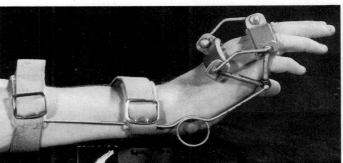

**Fig. 4.23** (a) Correction of the ulnar deformity (illustrated in Fig. 4.21a) by a neat lively splint. (b) The same patient wearing splint provided before arrival at the rehabilitation unit. It was unnecessarily clumsy and unattractive, and made dressing extremely difficult.

more effective than a continuous but minimal degree of physiotherapy.

Sensation in the ulnar distribution is regarded as far less important than that in the median, and this is relevant for the cutaneous supply. Reduced proprioception from an ulnar nerve lesion can be severely disabling, however; therefore exercises and functional movements should be given with this in mind. Activities should be designed to help maximise the sensory feedback, and typing and playing of those musical instruments that need finger control are particularly suitable. Speed can be gradually increased as ability improves. Support of the hand by resting the little finger on the table enables intricate movements of the thumb, index and middle fingers to be performed and this support is dependent on both cutaneous and proprioceptive feedback from the little finger. In the very early stages the patient must be warned not to let his anaesthetic little finger drop onto a hot iron etc. Localisation should be tested and retrained if necessary when sensation returns.

*Residual problems* of an ulnar nerve lesion, when regeneration is poor, include a permanent claw hand deformity affecting ring and little fingers. This may reduce the patient's ability to perform his work and leisure activities. Tendon transfers and other surgical techniques are designed to correct this deformity. If abductor digiti minimi recovers, but the interossei do not, the little finger may re-

main permanently abducted even when at rest, and can get in the way during functional activities (Fig. 4.24). This disability may also need to be corrected by surgery.

## Combined median and ulnar nerve lesions

When both median and ulnar nerves are involved the effects of each individual lesion combine to produce an extremely severe disability. The disability is more severe with the lesion at high level, when all the flexors of wrist and digits are affected and grasp becomes totally absent. It is inevitable that when both nerves are divided at wrist level there will also be tendon injuries, combined frequently with division of arteries and possibly joint capsule. The resulting scarring and fibrosis following bleeding will cause loss of tissue elasticity and the formation of adhesions between skin, tendons, nerves and sometimes the deeper structures of the joints. Ischaemia of the muscles may also occur following arterial damage.

The deformity that results is the totally flat claw hand (Fig. 4.25a & b). The intrinsic minus deformity will develop with gross hyperextension of the MCP joints if no support is given to prevent their over-mobility (Fig. 4.25c). This deformity can be extremely painful due to the stretch on capsule and ligaments. Forward thrust of fingers and thumb will be completely lost (Fig. 4.25d) and rolling flexion of the fingers will become pronounced. Sensation will be absent on the whole of the volar surface and over the dorsal surfaces of the tips of all fingers and the volar surface of the thumb. The autonomic effects will be visible in the same distribution, with a noticeable loss of pulp and subcutaneous tissue. Trick movements will be identical with those of the individual nerve lesions. Patients with combined lesions at high level, however, may be able to flex the wrist, although all the muscles considered to be wrist or finger flexors are paralysed. Flexion is possible because the tendon of abductor pollicis longus, with its radial nerve supply, lies immediately anterior to the fulcrum of the wrist joint. A tenodesis action is also demonstrated when the patient attempts to flex his fingers. The increased tension of the finger flexors produced by hyperextending the wrist will produce a small amount of passive finger flexion.

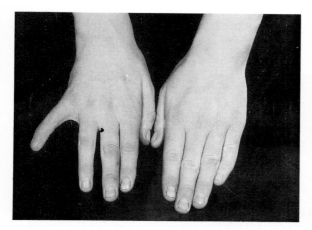

**Fig. 4.24** A residual problem of an ulnar nerve lesion. Adduction could be produced passively but not actively and the finger was continually getting caught. Surgery was necessary to correct this deformity.

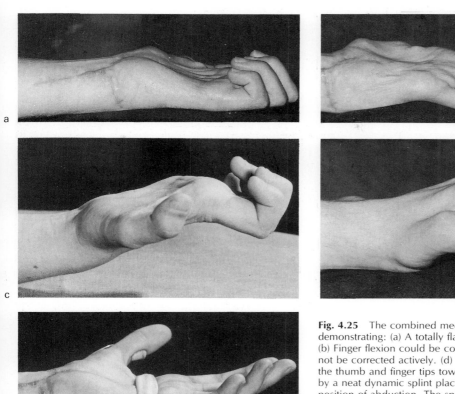
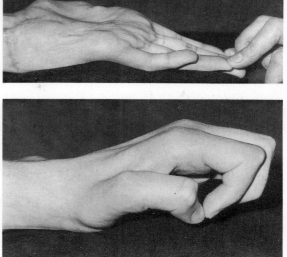

**Fig. 4.25** The combined median and ulnar nerve lesion demonstrating: (a) A totally flat hand with claw deformity. (b) Finger flexion could be corrected passively, (c) but could not be corrected actively. (d) Total inability to thrust forward the thumb and finger tips towards one another; (e) Correction by a neat dynamic splint placing the thumb in a functional position of abduction. The splint enabled the patient to extend his fingers for himself.

*Physiotherapy* is again involved with maintaining range of joints, elasticity of the soft tissues and an adequate circulation. Counselling and instruction on the care of the hand, especially of the anaesthetic areas, must be thorough. Lively splinting that prevents the deformity from becoming gross, enables the patient to extend his fingers and improves function should be arranged (Fig. 4.25e). Pain must also be treated before it becomes intractable.

It is the associated problems of fibrosis and adhesions of scarring, however, that will probably need the greatest intensity of treatment. The physiotherapist should be involved immediately after surgery in the elevation of the hand and arm to help prevent oedema, and in the movement of available joints and muscles, which will also ensure the best possible circulation in the limb.

Surgeons will have differing criteria for commencement of active movement, but delay after 3 weeks will allow tissues to become extremely fibrotic. Early activity, however, must be gentle and be increased gradually as too energetic a treatment will cause a renewed release of fibrinogen. Early passive stretching is totally contraindicated for this reason, besides putting an undesirable stretch on a sutured nerve. Further treatment for adherence of tendons is discussed on p. 164.

Intensity of treatment must again be increased when re-innervation occurs. It is unlikely that recovery can ever be total following such a severe injury and therefore it is imperative to maximise both motor and sensory functions. Repeated assessment of function is advisable over the following year. This applies particularly to sensory function as it is this more than poor motor function which is

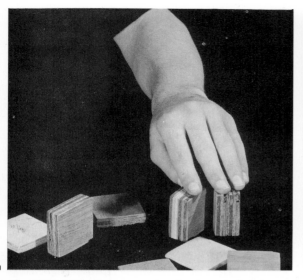
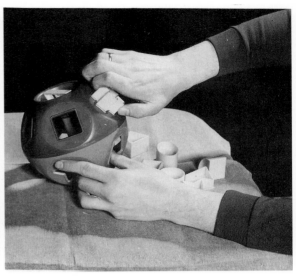

**Fig. 4.26(a & b)** Sensory re-education is particularly important during re-innervation of combined median and ulnar nerve lesions.

likely to prove the most disabling. Sessions of sensory training lasting a week or so every 3–4 months are found to be of greatest value until nerve recovery is complete (Fig. 4.26a & b).

*The residual problems* of combined lesions are the same as in the separate median and ulnar nerve lesions, further complicated by the greater degree of associated injuries. A gross hyperextension deformity of all four fingers may remain if re-innervation is poor, but this can be corrected by a superficialis transfer into the capsules of the MCP joints (Fig. 4.27a & b). Both flexor digitorum super-

ficialis and profundus must contract efficiently, however, before this procedure should be considered.

## Brachial plexus lesions

Lesions of the plexus, which are now quite commonly seen, are caused mainly by motor cycle or motor car accidents, but also by gun shot and stab wounds, compression from carrying a heavy pack and occasionally from malignancy and its treatment by radiotherapy. A traction injury can cause avulsion of the roots, with a resulting pre-ganglionic

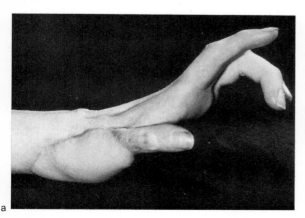
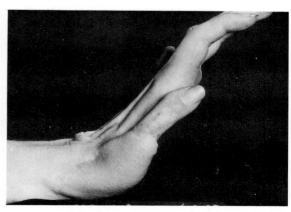

**Fig. 4.27** (a) Any residual clawing of the fingers as the result of poor re-innervation of the intrinsic muscles can cause a disability at work and during leisure hours. (b) Corrective surgery can produce excellent results.

lesion, and this is more serious than an injury caused by a direct blow at clavicular level when a post-ganglionic rupture or a lesion in continuity occurs. Varying combinations of lesions can occur, the most common being the C5 and C6 lesion. The totally flail arm that remains permanently paralysed is now becoming one of the more frequently seen injuries, due to the increasing speed at which accidents occur. Root lesions in isolation are rare.

The paralysis and loss of sensation resulting from a plexus lesion causes an extremely severe disability, especially when it involves the hand. Management by a team skilled in caring for these injuries is, therefore, absolutely essential. Diagnosing a disorder of such complexity requires conduction studies by electromyography (EMG), together with X-rays, spinograms (Jones 1979) and possible myelography. Normal sensory conduction on EMG indicates a pre-ganglionic lesion, as the posterior horn cell and the axons remain intact. Absence of sensory conduction leaves an unclear picture as the lesion may either be post-ganglionic or a combination of both pre- and post-ganglionic. Stimulation techniques performed by physiotherapists should not be used for diagnostic purposes. A good clinical assessment by the therapists, however, of the motor and sensory supply, of any residual function in the limb, and any problems such as pain or joint stiffness together with the patient's specific needs, forms an essential part of correct diagnosis and management.

Pre-ganglionic lesions have a bad prognosis as they cannot be repaired, they do not regenerate, and they are usually accompanied by severe pain. Post-ganglionic ruptures can possibly be repaired or grafted, axonotmeses may regenerate, and the pain is never so severe. Both good and bad prognostic signs are summarised by Wynn Parry (1981).

Early exploration of post-ganglionic lesions should be considered, to enable possible repair or grafting to be performed, together with repair of ruptured blood vessels. A definitive diagnosis can then be made, which should allow better management and the planning of later reconstructive procedures.

*Physiotherapy*, i.e. management and occasional short sessions of treatment, will be necessary over a period of several months.

Accurate motor and sensory assessment is es-

sential as it plays a big part in deciding the level of the lesion and in the total management of the patient. A rule-of-thumb guide which indicates the root level according to muscle activity is as follows:

C5 supplies deltoid, supraspinatus, infraspinatus rhomboids and other muscles of the shoulder region. If the rhomboids are not contracting the lesion is probably pre-ganglionic.

C6 supplies the flexors of the elbow, i.e. biceps, brachialis, and brachioradialis.

C7 supplies the extensors of the elbow, wrist and fingers.

C8 supplies the long flexors of wrist and fingers and usually the thenar muscles.

T1 supples the intrinsics, the hypothenar muscles and occasionally the thenar muscles. A Horner's syndrome is associated with a pre-ganglionic lesion at this level because of the sympathetic pathways between cervical ganglion and the eye. Constriction of the pupil is the most usual sign (Fig. 4.28a) combined with slight drooping of the eyelid.

N.B. Anomalies of root supply occur quite frequently, and it is possible for the plexus to be pre- or post-fixed.

When the lesion is extensive a sling must be worn to support the flail limb (Fig. 4.28b & c). The shoulder joint may sublux and become extremely painful if all the muscles that normally provide support are paralysed. The Williamson sling illustrated (Fig. 4.28d & e) was designed by the patient herself before seeing the Chessington version. It has pockets to hold money, make-up and cigarettes, etc. and can be made in a variety of colours. The reverse picture shows an additional strap passing over the top of the shoulder and under the elbow which supports the glenohumeral joint, thus preventing subluxation.

Periodic assessment should be carried out to discover any recovering muscle activity in order to maximise function by re-education. Sensation should also be charted for normal, anaesthetic and altered sensory areas. It should be remembered that the dermatomes from root distribution will be totally different from the peripheral nerve sensory pattern.

The physiotherapist's role following a plexus

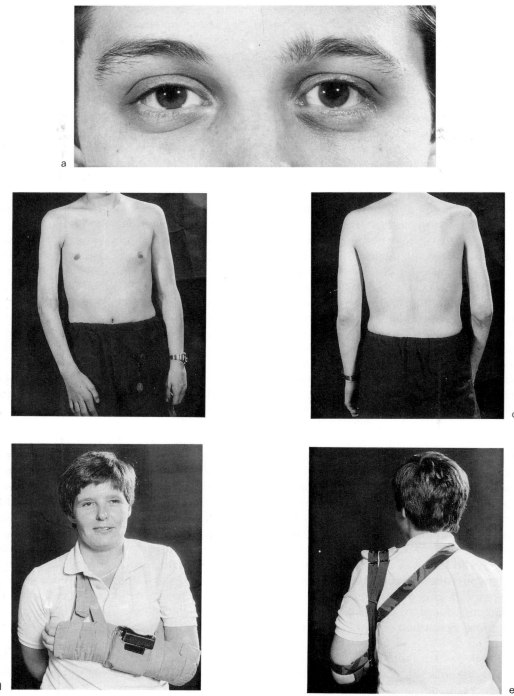

**Fig. 4.28** (a) A Horner's syndrome as the result of a brachial plexus lesion demonstrates constriction of the pupil and slight drooping of the eyelid. (b & c) Typical posture and wasting of a plexus lesion patient. The upper arm is internally rotated and the forearm is pronated. On examination note the difference in colour, the flat hand and thumb and the extended fingers. (d) The Williamson sling designed by the patient herself, with pockets for possessions. (e) An additional strap with pad over the affected shoulder supports the glemo-humeral joint.

lesion, besides assessing the patient, is mainly to teach him how to manage his limb for himself. Joint and web space mobility and muscle extensibility must be maintained by full range passive movements of the arm and hand. Special emphasis should be put on metacarpophalangeal joint flexion, on maintaining the webs, on external rotation together with abduction of the shoulder, and supination of the forearm together with elbow extension, as these rotatory movements can stiffen rapidly. Associated injuries such as fractures may produce a joint stiffness that is difficult to correct in a paralysed limb. Some patients will have discovered the passive movements for themselves while others will need tuition.

Pain can frequently be the main problem as far as the patient is concerned. TNS should be tried, although with root avulsion it is less likely to be successful. The electrodes must be placed on skin with sensation, and therefore to be effective when there is extensive sensory loss they may need to be positioned over the same dermatomes on the contralateral side. Sufficient time must be allowed and variations of position tried in order to produce a satisfactory effect. This can best be achieved in conjunction with well-kept records of the level of pain before and after treatment, the position of the electrodes and the dosage given.

Unless there is a special need for treatment of joint stiffness or pain, patients should not, in the early stages, require regular physiotherapy. They will, however, need sufficient counselling so that they can understand the nature and effects of the injury, and know that their work and social problems are cared for. Most plexus lesions take months or even a year or so to achieve the best functional result, be it very little. It is therefore essential that the patient can feel that support and the best advice are available. Some like to learn about the level of the lesion and the muscles affected, and this helps to ensure that the patient takes a good interest in his limb and watches for any recovery.

It is important psychologically that the patient should, if at all possible, return to work. This may mean performing a modified or totally altered role. A splint for the flail arm should help the patient to perform tasks that require the use of both limbs. Suitable tools for both work and leisure interests can be attached (Wynn Parry 1984). The patient learns to use the splint in the occupational therapy department and workshops.

Re-education should commence immediately any recovery of muscle activity is seen in order to maximise function. Short bursts are found to be better than continuous treatment, as the patient himself must practise the exercises at home. Recovering sensation in the hand will probably need sessions of formal re-education. Incorrect localisation, due to crossed reinnervation, may develop but can be improved with sensory training.

Co-contraction of muscles occasionally occurs, due also to crossed re-innervation, and is a problem that can be difficult to correct. The patient is unable to prevent a simultaneous contraction of agonist and antagonist, with the result that antigravity movements may be impossible to achieve. The power and bulk of the muscles, however, may appear to be building up well. The most common examples are:

1. Co-contraction of biceps and triceps. Gravity plus contraction of triceps can negate any elbow flexion.
2. Co-contraction of deltoid and pectoralis major. Elevation of the shoulder using deltoid may be prevented by the simultaneous contraction of pectoralis major, together with the effect of gravity.

Observation of muscles during their early recovery and careful retraining is therefore essential if co-contraction is suspected. Muscles must learn not only to contract but also to relax at the appropriate moment. Movements which will activate the one muscle into inner range, and which should therefore produce reflex relaxation of the antagonist in its outer range, should be practised. Pendular movements and sling suspension are most useful in the initial stage. Biofeedback, preferably using a reciprocal apparatus and EMG electrodes, should help the patient learn to relax his antagonist muscles, but it is a difficult problem for some to correct. More functional activities can be introduced when the relaxation control improves. Reversing the origin and insertion of muscles in pushing movements and in body support are also of value.

### Later stages after plexus lesions

Residual disabilities due to non-recovery of a plexus

lesion can sometimes be improved by reconstructive surgery. The therapists play an essential role at this stage with their assessment of joints and muscles (including power in the non-affected muscles) and sensation of the limb, of any functional activities that the patient can perform using the affected arm, and of his ability to manage with only one normal hand and arm. If after a year or so the patient manages perfectly well it may be that surgical procedures are not indicated. If, however, he badly needs the return of some function, e.g. elbow flexion, careful consideration of this must be given, preferably by a team of specialists. The transfer of muscles can sometimes have a surprising and, in some instances, disastrous effect for an already disabled patient.

Unaffected or recovered muscles may be used as donors for tendon transfer procedures. They may be weak following either disuse or little use of the limb, and if below grade 4 are unsuitable as donors. Occasionally it is necessary to arthrodese a joint in order to provide stability but this should only ever apply to the glenohumeral joint and the wrist joint.

Reconstructive surgery in brachial plexus lesions is more complicated than in peripheral nerve injuries (Frampton 1986). Mobility of joints, power of muscle donors, loss of cutaneous sensation and proprioception must be successfully treated prior to operation. Post-operatively the patient is likely to need some intensive physiotherapy before he can achieve an adequate contraction of the transfer (see p. 167).

Amputation may need to be considered for extensive non-recovery of a flail arm. It is less frequently recommended these days, and a high proportion of patients in the past have not worn their prostheses. It must obviously only be contemplated after diagnostic tests have been made by specialists and non-recovery is absolutely certain.

The flail limb of a plexus patient can hinder both work and leisure activities and can possibly be dangerous in some occupations, especially when totally anaesthetic. The hand may easily be burnt or otherwise injured and may take a long time to heal. It can also become very swollen and discoloured and hence be rather unsightly. Some patients are therefore keen to have the limb or hand amputated. They must be in a position to

sum up the advantages and disadvantages and finally make a decision for themselves. Many find that the use of the flail arm splint is preferable to making such an irrevocable decision.

Factors to be considered include:
1. Provision of stability and control of the shoulder is essential for using a prosthesis. Arthrodesis may be necessary if the glenohumeral joint is flail, thereby enabling some shoulder girdle control. For a below-elbow amputation there must be some active elbow flexion, either already present or from possible tendon transfer. These procedures are liable to take several months to carry out.
2. The patient must consider not only the advantages that a prosthesis can give in employment and leisure activities but also the psychological effect from the loss of the hand and the reaction of the public. He must realise, if he suffers pain in his hand or limb, that amputation will not remove that pain. Pain in a phantom limb is most likely and this will be even more frustrating than experiencing pain in a hand that is still present.

## TENDON INJURIES

Tendon injuries, and even those of seemingly minor involvement, can result in a severe disability, and therefore require skilful management. Rest, which is necessary to promote healing after surgery, conflicts with the need to mobilise in order to prevent the formation of adhesions. An increase in the number of criss-cross sutures that should be used may, in the future, provide a stronger repair, thereby allowing early mobilisation to be performed with safety (Savage 1985).

Normal excursion of the flexor tendons, from full finger extension to full finger flexion, is approximately 3.0–4.0 cm in profundus but slightly less in superficialis. Flexion of the distal joint accounts for the extra excursion of profundus and also is responsible for the gliding that occurs between profundus and superficialis (McGrouther & Ahmed 1981). There is less excursion of the extensor tendons over the dorsum of the hand.

Tendons are divided mainly as a result of lacerations from knives or glass, from road accidents and severe crushing injuries and occasionally from ruptures at the insertion. The final functional result is better following a clean division of one tendon only than after the involvement of several tendons and other structures, with possible haematoma formation and infection from dirty wounds, and combined with loss of sensation.

Results also depend largely on the site of injury. Flexor tendon injuries have been classified into zones by Verdan (1960) (Fig. 4.29).

*Zone 1* is distal to the insertion of superficialis, therefore affects profundus only.

*Zone 2* or 'No man's land' (Bunnell 1970) is the section where the fibrous sheath is occupied by both superficialis and profundus. This is mainly in the finger but is partly in the distal section of the palm also.

*Zone 3* is the palmar section where the fibrous sheath is absent.

*Zone 4* is under the carpal tunnel.

*Zone 5* is at the wrist, proximal to the carpal tunnel. Frequently several tendons are divided and nerves are involved.

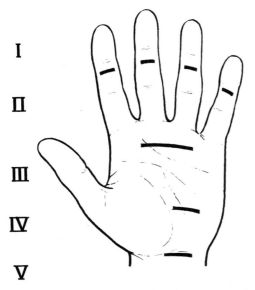

**Fig. 4.29** Zones for classification of tendon injuries in the hand.

## Tendon repair

A primary tendon repair should be performed whenever possible in order to achieve the best results. The located tendon ends are held by trans-fixing needles so that the repair can be performed in the absence of tension (Smith & Boardman 1986). The two strands of a criss-cross suture approximate and hold the ends of the tendon while the peripheral (circumferential) suture ensures a smooth exterior to the repair. Pulleys, if damaged, should be repaired if possible to prevent later bow-stringing of the tendons.

Tendons receive a large part of their blood supply from the surrounding tissues so that adequate time must be given to ensure the viability of the repair before any force can be applied. Tension should be totally relieved by the use of some form of splintage for the first few weeks.

Division of either one or both the flexor tendons in *zone 2*, or 'no man's land' demands the best surgical expertise. In the past the results of primary suture were poor, mainly because the suture material formed a bulky repair and this was unable to glide in the restricted space of the tendon sheath. Nowadays, with the use of the microscope together with the extremely fine suturing materials available, the improved quality of surgery fully justifies a primary repair in 'no man's land'.

Following the repair a dorsal back-slab is applied, shaped so that the wrist is held in approximately 30° flexion and the MCP joints in 90° flexion. The distal section of the splint should be straight to allow the IP joints to extend fully when exercised (Fig. 4.30a). With the hand resting in the splint the affected finger is pulled into flexion by a rubber band which is attached by a loop of thread through the tip of the finger nail (Fig. 4.30b). The other end of the band is then attached just proximal to the wrist, in line with the scaphoid. This is the Kleinert dynamic splintage (Kleinert et al 1973) which takes the tension off the sutured tendon while allowing it to be freely mobilised.

Some surgeons prefer to place all the fingers in this dynamic splintage. It prevents any possible chance of damage occurring to the repair if the patient uses his unaffected fingers. The contracting muscle belly activates the tendons to all the fingers, and a rupture of the repair has occasionally resulted.

A modification of this Kleinert splint can be made by placing a thick wire across the palm to act as a pulley (Slattery & McGrouther 1984). The wire is first threaded through a fine rubber tube before the ends are fixed into the back slab. The

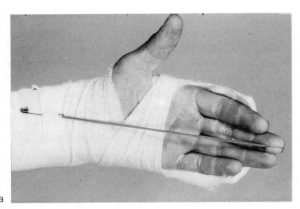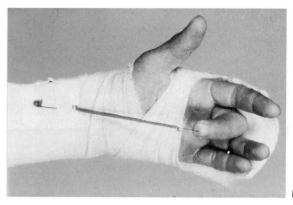

**Fig. 4.30(a & b)**   Kleinert dynamic splintage demonstrates active extension and passive flexion of the interphalangeal joints.

rubber band attached to the finger nail is passed under the wire and the rubber tube acts as a roller to eliminate friction. A greater range of flexion is produced in the distal interphalangeal joint by this modification. Not all surgeons, however, use this dynamic splintage method; some prefer to rest the tendon and maintain mobility by passive flexion of the finger. Only after 3 weeks is active movement introduced.

Division of several tendons in *zone 5* at the wrist usually involves nerves also. Care has to be taken to identify the proximal and distal ends of the divided tendons for correct approximation, and mistakes are not totally unknown.

A secondary tendon repair is the procedure performed either when a primary repair has failed or when there has been a considerable delay between injury and surgery. This delay may be necessary if the surrounding tissues have been severely trauma-

tised and have become infected. Healing is necessary before tendon surgery can be considered.

### Tendon graft

In zone 2, or 'no man's land' a secondary repair is by tendon graft (Fig. 4.32 a & b). Palmaris longus is the most frequently used donor tendon when it is present in the ipsilateral limb. An extensor tendon to a toe or the plantaris tendon may otherwise be used.

If the site for the graft is scarred and fibrosed a silastic rod is sometimes inserted and attached at either end to the profundus tendon for 3–4 weeks immediately prior to the graft. A smooth bed is formed by the passive gliding motion of the rod in the finger. It must not be used actively. The graft is then positioned without the need to re-open the finger as it is attached to the proximal end of the

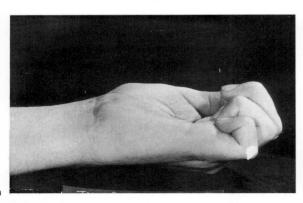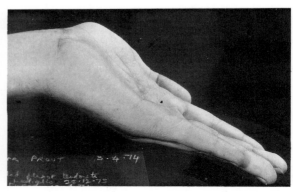

**Fig. 4.31(a & b)**   Result following the primary suture of divided tendons to the middle finger. Dynamic splintage was not used for this patient.

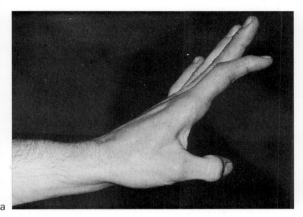
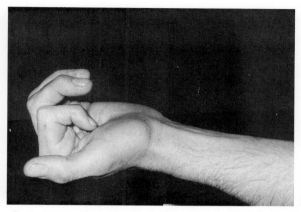

a
b

**Fig. 4.32(a & b)**   Result of a palmaris longus graft to the middle finger showing slight reduction of extension, but excellent finger flexion.

rod, and the rod is pulled through from the distal end, carrying the new graft with it. It is sutured into position in place of the rod. The hand and fingers are usually rested for 3 weeks in a plaster slab.

A graft is dependent on receiving its blood supply from the surrounding tissues, which is why rest is most usual. Kleinert splintage is occasionally used when conditions are particularly advantageous.

### Physiotherapy

Loss of passive range as well as active movement may occur with a delay prior to tendon repair. It is essential, before surgery, that a full range is regained in those joints affected by the tendon or the repair is unlikely to succeed. Mobilisation by active and accessory movements, passive stretches and stretch splinting should be given intensively until full mobility is achieved.

Measurements that include both the range of the affected joints and the excursion of the digit or the whole hand and wrist, whichever is appropriate, should be made as early as possible after surgery. The flexion and extension deficit (Smith & Boardman 1986) is a suitable measure of the movement in a finger. The position in which the joints are at rest should also be measured: this may be identical to the fully flexed position. If this is the case any adherence is totally blocking active flexion and will therefore need special attention.

Physiotherapy following surgery is usually necessary for the prevention or treatment of the following:

### 1. Oedema

Elevation both when the patient is in bed and when ambulant will usually prevent oedema from becoming a problem.

### 2. Adhesions

Adhesions are liable to form between the repaired tendon, its sheath, the lacerated skin and the surrounding tissues unless preventative measures can be taken. Use of the dynamic Kleinert splint is an effective means of preventing this adherence following primary repairs in zones 1, 2 and 3.

### 3. Joint stiffness

If adhesions are allowed to form around the repaired tendon they will inevitably have an effect on the joints, sometimes severely limiting range of movement. Inner range may be maintained passively, as it puts no tension on the repair. Outer range, however, may remain limited until the adhesions are freed. As this sometimes takes several weeks a contracture of both ligaments and capsule may result. This is another reason why the problem of adhesions should receive prompt attention.

The adherence usually has a primary effect on the joint in closest proximity and a secondary effect on those joints distal to the repair. For example, a laceration of tendons at the wrist, with both wrist and fingers immobilised in some degree of flexion, will frequently produce adhesions at the wrist.

This will mainly limit wrist extension but to a lesser extent wrist flexion also. The effect on the more distal joints is to limit the simultaneous extension of the fingers. However, each distal joint can be mobilised individually without any strain being put on the repair. The slackening of tension at the other joints will allow the selected joint to be moved easily through its full passive range.

### 4. Incorrect or lost movement patterns

Patients may have lost the correct feeling of movement, particularly when there is sensory nerve involvement combined with tendon injury. It is important that a digital nerve, for instance, is repaired together with the tendon following injury to a finger.

A considerable delay between tendon injury and repair may have allowed the patient to develop a habit of altered movement. After a division of flexors digitorum profundus and superficialis, for instance, the only finger flexion is at the MCP joints, performed by the intrinsic muscles. These muscles also extend the IP joints, which is the direct opposite of the action required from the repaired FDP and FDS. Any altered movement will therefore need careful re-education.

### Adhesions

Adhesions that form around a tendon following repair are severely disabling and present an enormous challenge to the physiotherapist. Some patients are unfortunate in that they react to surgery by producing a vast amount of fibrous tissue. The need for dynamic splintage is most applicable for this type of patient, but when it is not suitable the tendon must be immobilised by a resting splint for 3 weeks.

Massage using hydrous ointment a few days after surgery will help to soften any induration of tissues around the scar. Ultrasonics treatment is contra-indicated for 4 weeks, as it has been shown to delay tendon healing (Roberts et al 1982).

Deep frictional-type massage, using a little lanolin to prevent damage to the skin, should be used to stretch any adhesions that have already formed. After 4–5 weeks a better effect can be achieved by giving this massage with the tendon on tension than with it relaxed, when skin, tendon and underlying tissues shift as one under the therapist's fingers. Firstly, the patient should actively flex the finger, or appropriate joint, and hold the position whilst the frictional massage is given immediately over and around the tendon. In particular it should be applied in a caudal direction.

Secondly, the massage is repeated while the patient actively extends his finger and then holds the position. Thirdly, when it is safe to apply a passive stretch, the finger or hand should be stretched into maximum extension by the physiotherapist, who again applies massage over the tensioned tendon. During the latter two instances, the concentration of massage should be in a cephalad direction.

Pressure applied by the physiotherapist can also enable the patient to stretch any adhesions between skin and tendons actively for himself. This applies especially where the skin is very mobile, e.g. over the flexor aspect of the wrist. The physiotherapist's firm pressure should be applied on the skin immediately proximal to the scar, and the patient actively flexes either wrist or fingers or both as appropriate. The exercise is then reversed with the pressure applied, wherever possible, distal to the scar, and the patient actively extends his wrist and fingers. The physiotherapist attempts, in both directions, to prevent the adherent scar from sliding under her fingers. This can be an uncomfortable exercise so should be performed cautiously at first.

When the tendon repair is sound, vigorous exercises should be given, with repeated stretch applied by the physiotherapist to the contracting muscles. Resisted movements to the antagonists, passive stretching, and lively or stretch splinting may all help to free adhesions. This passive stretching of adhesions, which is possible in one direction only, can have the effect of improving active movement in both directions. Frequent monitoring by the therapist is necessary of both excursion and range of movement, and of the position at rest, so that instant adjustment of treatment can be made, as a gain in one direction may undesirably be at the expense of movement in the opposite direction.

*Priorities* for recovering movements are as follows:

1. With adherence of the flexor tendons the first priority is to regain active flexion, as this can only be achieved by the patient's own active work.

Extension is easier to recover because passive stretching and splinting can also be used to achieve movement.

Therapist and patient should therefore concentrate on improving flexion and maintaining extension. Once the flexion has improved, more emphasis can be put on recovering extension, while ensuring that no flexion is lost.

2. With adherence of the extensor tendons the priority is to regain extension by active movement. The active power of the flexors is usually sufficient to stretch and mobilise any adherent scar on the dorsum of the hand and wrist.

It is important that the hand is immobilised with the divided tendons in approximately a middle to outer range position when Kleinert suspension is not used. Never should the tendons be positioned in total outer range as there is then little chance of stretching any adhesions and the patient has the daunting task ahead of him of trying to regain full range by active movement only.

*Following the primary suture of flexor tendons in zones 1, 2, and 3* it is safe to commence physiotherapy immediately when dynamic Kleinert splinting is used. The patient is asked to extend against the rubber band until the dorsum of his finger rests against the back-slab. It may be necessary to urge him into this full extension, making repeated attempts until the movement is performed easily.

Reflex reciprocal relaxation of the flexors occurs during active extension of the fingers against resistance. Having achieved full extension the extensors are relaxed, thereby allowing the elastic band to flex the finger passively. Thus very little tension is applied at any time to the repaired tendon. Healing is slightly slower, however, when using this Kleinert suspension than when the tendon is rested completely. The traction therefore remains on the finger for 4–5 weeks, i.e. 2 weeks longer than for a totally rested tendon.

It is important to check that the patient performs the correct movement several times a day for himself and that the plaster back-slab is shaped so that it allows full IP joint extension, yet maintains the MCP joints in flexion. The patient should be repeatedly warned not to use his other fingers for activities requiring any degree of power. The contraction of the muscle belly has been known to rupture the repair, even when that particular finger was not being used. The other fingers should therefore be placed in Kleinert suspension also, if it is thought that the patient might be careless.

Free active flexion can be commenced when the traction and back-slab have been removed. There should be no joint stiffness if the post-operative regime has been diligent, and a good pull through of the flexors is usually possible, indicating that no adhesions have formed. Graduated resistance is introduced at 7–8 weeks and the patient should have returned to a normal existence within 2½ months of injury.

*Following a primary repair at the wrist (zone 5),* where both tendons and nerves are frequently divided, the whole hand is usually rested by a dorsal slab for 3 weeks. Kleinert suspension, if applied to the fingers when both nerves and tendons have been divided at the wrist, prevents any active movement of the wrist until approximately 5 weeks after surgery. Many surgeons therefore prefer to immobilise all divided structures for 3 weeks, at which time active movement may be safely commenced.

Gentle free active movement of wrist and finger flexors should be given. Extension should be tried cautiously at first, in order not to stretch any nerve suture. Regaining the flexion movements of the fingers must be the first priority whilst ensuring that extension is not lost. If extension decreases a light volar resting splint can be used at night, but a stretch should not be applied at this stage. Extension of the wrist should be combined with flexion of the fingers at first (Fig. 4.33a).

Graduated resistance can be introduced at 5–6 weeks after surgery and passive stretching, if it is necessary, at 8 weeks. Stretch splinting is safe after 9–10 weeks, but should only be used if the patient's range is not being increased by more conservative methods (Fig. 4.33b).

Intensive rehabilitation with increasing activity is essential when there is much scarring and adhesion formation in this zone. It is particularly necessary if nerves are also divided. Full joint range and tendon function must be regained quickly in order that motor and sensory re-education can be commenced, as soon as reinnervation occurs, on a mobile hand.

*Following a graft in zone 2* when the tendon has

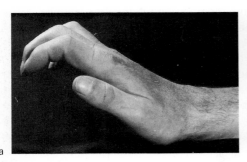
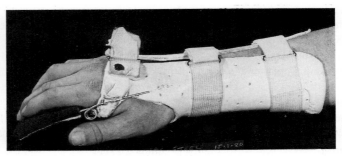

**Fig. 4.33** (a) Inability to fully extend his IP joints handicapped this patient. (b) A strong lively splint stretched the contracture and this fireman returned to duty.

been totally immobilised, physiotherapy may be commenced at three weeks. The range of movement should be measured: the position of joints at rest, the actively flexed and extended positions, and also the passive flexion should be recorded. Passive extension must not be attempted at this stage.

The scar will usually have healed by this time and a warm soak followed by massage with a hydrous ointment will help both to remove any dead skin that may have accumulated and to soften any adhesions. Passive flexion movements should be given to ensure a full flexion range, but not passive extension.

The range of movement of the interphalangeal joints is frequently rather limited following grafting because of the adhesions that form. The patient may have difficulty in learning to contract flexor digitorum profundus in isolation. His attempt to flex the finger will automatically include flexion of the MCP joint. If the IP joints are observed carefully they will frequently be seen to shoot into a fully extended position, although the patient is still attempting to flex his finger. This is because he is using the intrinsic muscles which act not only as flexors of the MCP joint but also as extensors of the IP joints. The IP joints are thus actively splinted in extension so strongly that the weak FDP is unable to produce any movement at all. It is therefore essential that the patient learns to contract FDP, and also FDS if still present, without the intrinsic muscles working.

With the dorsum of both hands on the pillow the patient must first practise contracting in isolation the long flexors of all the normal fingers. This will produce a clawing action, with the MCP joints

remaining in extension. Having got the feel of the correct performance of this movement, the patient should then attempt to reproduce it in his affected finger, using only very gentle and extremely small range free active contractions. Any small movement that is detected at the correct joint should be pointed out immediately. Support should not be given over the proximal phalanx at this stage because the patient is likely to flex his MCP joint against the support and thus oppose the desired movement. Free active extension exercises should also be given.

At 5–6 weeks, when the correct activity is clearly improving, resistance may be added gradually and activities introduced which involve all the joints of the whole hand. By 8–9 weeks all strong movements should be safe. If necessary, passive stretching and stretch splints may then be used to improve the extension range.

The re-education of tendon grafts is usually rather tedious from the patient's point of view. The more intelligent he is the more frustrating he finds the inevitable slow progress, with little obvious sign that he is improving at all. A few degrees of extra range a week is quite acceptable, however, and this should be pointed out when the measurements are taken. The patient who can sit quietly and flex and extend his finger repetitively is the one who is most likely to recover maximum function.

### Complications of tendon injuries

The main complication for the physiotherapist following tendon repair is the presence of adhesions. If after several weeks of intensive treatment, which includes passive stretching and stretch and lively splinting, the adhesions have still not improved, surgery may be necessary. Stretch may start to produce pain in the joints because the joint surfaces are being compressed. At this stage the range should be maintained without using the extreme stretch procedures that cause pain. Many surgeons prefer to delay a tenolysis for 6 months to prevent an exacerbation of scar tissue.

## TENDON TRANSFERS

Transfers may be performed following the non-recovery of a peripheral nerve or cervical cord lesion in order to return active function to the hand or limb and to correct any persistent deformities that result. They may also be performed after tendon division or rupture, with the inherent repair difficulties (Fig. 4.34a & b) and for ischaemic contractures or muscle necrosis.

With extensive and permanent paralysis it may be necessary to arthrodese the wrist joint also. This then allows the donor tendons to return some movement to the fingers and thumb. It is difficult in fact for the patient to learn to control combined wrist and finger movements if only one donor is provided.

At operation, the distal end of the donor tendon is divided, repositioned and sutured to the receptor tendon. Occasionally the whole donor muscle together with its neurovascular supply is repositioned to a new site of origin before the distal tendon suture is performed. This procedure is used to improve the direction of muscle activity when in its new position.

A large variety of transfers can now be performed, but the most commonly used for the hand are those that return extension function following a radial nerve lesion and the transfer that returns opposition to the thumb following a median nerve lesion.

The effects of the transfers must be given careful thought as the donor loses 1 grade (Oxford Scale) when repositioned. It therefore must be at least grade 4 and preferably 5 before transfer. Loss of power from the donor's original position must also be considered. The transfer of a muscle essential to some important activity can produce a disastrous result for an already disabled person. It must therefore be given very careful prior consideration.

*Physiotherapy* for tendon transfers should include a complete assessment of the patient prior to the decision to operate. Examination of the affected muscles, the power of the suggested donors and the range of all joints, should be thorough. Sensation should also be charted together with any areas of incorrect localisation. What the patient finds difficult and what activities he would like to perform following transfers should be ascertained. Unless he is well motivated and has reasonably good sensation he will be unlikely to use his hand and arm.

The joints must be mobile prior to surgery. This may sometimes need several weeks of intensive treatment to achieve. It is also important that the patient can isolate or at least identify the donor muscle's contraction as it will greatly facilitate the post-operative re-education.

Following the operation the hand or limb will probably be immobilised for 2–3 weeks, during which time the free joints must be kept mobile and available muscles exercised. Occasionally the surgeon permits gentle re-education after 1 week only. When the immobilising splint has been removed, the transferred muscle should be re-educated with gravity eliminated at first. Usually the patient learns the desired movement remarkably easily. This is probably due to the fact that the motor unit has a particularly low ratio of nerve to muscle fibres, which enables especially good neuromuscular control.

Re-education of transfers for brachial plexus lesions is not so spontaneous as for peripheral nerve lesions due to a variety of factors (Frampton 1986), and they will need longer and more intensive sessions of treatment. When difficulty is experienced, some time should be spent identifying a contraction of the donor muscle, and comparing it with the same muscle and normal movement of the contralateral limb. The patient is then told to think both of the movement which the donor normally makes together with the desired new movement. These movements may appear to conflict, e.g. flexor carpi ulnaris may have been transferred into extensor digitorum following a radial nerve lesion. As the patient is attempting to extend the fingers using the new transfer it is undesirable to think of flexing the wrist in order to activate the donor muscle. It is, however, pertinent to think of deviating the wrist in an ulnar direction at the same time as extending the fingers.

When the transfer is from one aspect of the forearm to the other the tendons may be taken through the interosseous membrane, but some may be better passed subcutaneously (Birch & Grant 1986). In this case the muscle bellies or tendons can usually be identified as they wind obliquely round the ulna or radius. Gentle tapping or pressure applied by the therapist's hand, and when necessary icing, brushing and electrical stimulation of those muscles, may help the patient who has difficulty in regaining a correct contraction and thereby a new movement. Biofeedback may also be useful, using EMG electrodes placed on the donor, which allows the patient to observe on the screen his correct muscle contraction.

Active movement will be of small amplitude at first and probably in the middle of range. The primary aim should be to increase the active movement into inner range. Only when this active inner range is improving should the outer range be increased.

Gravity must not be allowed to stretch the muscle into outer range, and the hand, limb or digit must therefore be supported at first by the therapist's hands when exercising and by a splint or a sling as appropriate. Outer range is best regained by increasing the activity of the antagonists in preference to stretching passively.

*Tendon transfers most commonly used to improve hand function*

1. For non-recovery of a radial nerve lesion pronator teres, flexor carpi ulnaris and palmaris longus (if present) are used for restoring wrist extension, finger and thumb extension, and thumb abduction respectively (Fig. 4.35a & b).

2. For non-recovery in a median nerve lesion an opponens transfer is performed to restore opposition and palmar abduction of the thumb (Fig. 4.36a). The tendon of FDS to the ring finger is detached at insertion, retracted and passed through a loop that has been formed using a section of the FCU at its insertion. The tendon of FDS is passed under the thenar muscles and sutured into the dorsal expansion of the MCP joint of the thumb. This position of insertion is vital as it ensures that the thumb not only abducts but rotates also (Fig. 4.36b & c). Re-education is helped if the patient thinks of flexing the PIP joint of the ring finger, and at the same time gently abducts his thumb in a palmar direction.

This operation will only succeed when sensation in the thumb is near to normal.

3. For non-recovery of an ulnar nerve lesion, if the claw deformity is pronounced, a Zancolli 'lasso' procedure may be performed using FDS of at least grade 4 (see Fig. 4.27a & b). FDS tendon is detached from its insertion and is sutured back on itself, remaining 'lassoed' through the flexor sheath pulley at the level of the MCP joint. When the FDS contracts it pulls on the pulley, thus actively flexing the MCP joint and preventing it from hyperextending.

A permanently abducted little finger caused by the non-recovery of the palmar interosseous to that finger can be corrected by plication of the capsule of the MCP joint. Extreme weakness of pinch grip can be improved by transferring extensor indicis to the first dorsal interosseous.

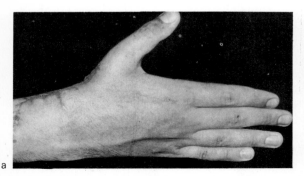
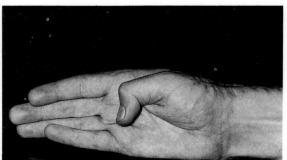

**Fig. 4.34(a & b)** Tendon transfer of extensor carpi radialis brevis following division of extensor pollicis longus.

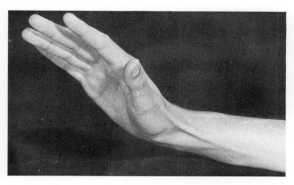

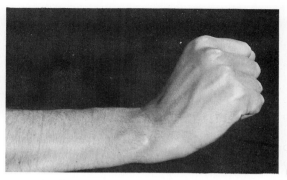

**Fig. 4.35(a & b)** The excellent result from transfer following a radial nerve lesion enabled this policeman to return to normal duty.

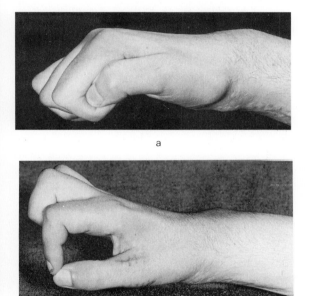

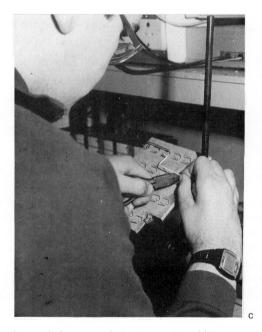

**Fig. 4.36** (a) The poor position of this patient's thumb following a median and ulnar nerve lesion incapacitated him considerably. (b) An opponens transfer much improved his function. (c) He was able to return to his interrupted training as a technician.

## Problems

Tension of the transferred tendon is crucial. If it is too slack, the donor muscle will be unable to activate inner range movement. Movement can improve with several months of exercising as the muscle has a contractile property. Shortening by surgery, however, may eventually be advisable. If the tension is too tight it will prevent movement into full outer range. Again this may improve with time, as the muscle belly is an elastic mechanism. Surgery to correct the tension when too tight may also need to be considered. The transferred tendon may not always effect the desired movement because of its direction of pull. If the muscle passes over more than one flail joint it may be unable to control the proximal joints. All likely effects must be considered carefully prior to surgery as they will be difficult to correct later.

## Tenolysis

Tenolysis, or the surgical excision of adhesions that surround and restrict the movements of tendons, may be necessary if range of movement does not increase and function remains reduced. If both active and passive stretching of the adherence causes pain in a joint, especially after intensive treatment has been given, it is unlikely that the adhesions will become freed without surgical intervention; but the surgeons are unlikely to perform a tenolysis until 6 months after injury in order to limit any exacerbation of fibrosis.

*Post-operative physiotherapy* must be commenced early, usually the day after surgery. Exercises given must be gentle at first because the excision of adhesions may have reduced the blood supply to the tendon, leaving it vulnerable to excess stress.

The patient is encouraged to exercise through as large a range as possible, so that full movement is achieved within a few days. Pain killers may be necessary initially if the movements are extremely uncomfortable. Power can be built up gradually after 2–3 weeks.

## Tenosynovitis and tenovaginitis

Tenosynovitis is an inflammatory condition of the synovial lining of the tendon sheaths resulting from injury. An increased amount of synovial fluid is secreted so that a swelling along the length of the sheath results. It may follow either mild trauma or some unaccustomed hard work of the hand and wrist. Occasionally it follows a penetration of the synovium by, for instance, a thorn, when it is liable to become infected. It also frequently results from rheumatoid arthritis.

Tenovaginitis describes the condition when there is a painful and hard thickening of the synovium without excessive synovial fluid secretion. It can be palpated along the affected tendon sheath. It is commonly experienced as the result of repetitive and stressful work. In recent years, for instance, it has become an occupational hazard for those working in poultry processing factories.

Abductor pollicis longus and extensors pollicis longus and brevis are the tendons most commonly affected by persistent or unaccustomed trauma. Pain and crepitus are experienced on movement

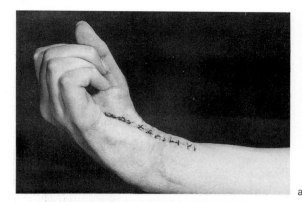

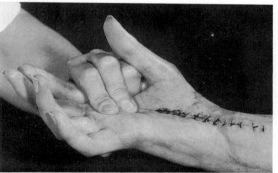

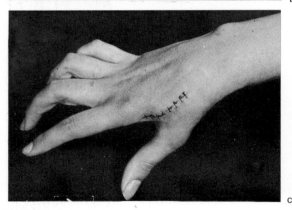

**Fig. 4.37(a, b & c)** Active movements given to a patient a few days after extensive resection of fibrotic tissue in the thumb web and tenolysis of the flexor tendons. This surgery followed 9 months after a median and ulnar nerve lesion, the division of tendons and severe ischaemic damage from a road traffic accident.

and if the condition is infected or acute it may be painful at rest also.

An infected synovial sheath must be dealt with urgently by surgery, irrigation and the introduction of antibiotics. Necrosis of the tendon may otherwise result (Wilson 1983).

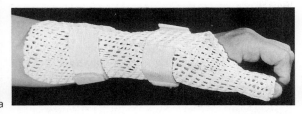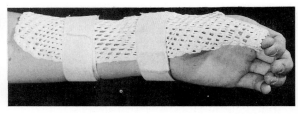

a                                                                                  b

**Fig. 4.38(a & b)** Splint support for the thumb affected by tenovaginitis of EPL and APB. Note that some function is possible by contact of index finger to the thumb tip.

Rest is the most important aspect of conservative treatment. Support with a crepe bandage or splint may be adequate, but frequently a cylinder which provides complete immobilisation is essential. Hexcelite is a suitable material to use as it is both rigid and aerated. PEMF helps to reduce pain and swelling, and can be given through bandages or plaster of Paris. Resistant small areas can be massaged using ice cubes. Ultrasound, which is usually given with the splint removed, is found to be more effective if the condition has already become chronic. One or two treatments of low dosage continuous ultrasound, or frictions, over the painful area, may temporarily exacerbate the symptoms and should be followed by some pulsed treatments. This technique has been more effective than other methods when the condition has become chronic. A localised painful spot can often be cured finally by a hydrocortisone injection. Exercise should then be introduced gradually to build up normal muscle power.

Surgery may be necessary if the condition is totally resistant to conservative treatment. An incision of the sheath relieves the pressure on the tendon, and very gentle exercises can be introduced 4–5 days later. It is very important to prevent adhesions from forming.

*Trigger finger*, with the nodular thickening of a flexor tendon, may also need an incision of the sheath when conservative treatment methods have failed, in order to allow normal tendon gliding.

Measures may have to be taken to prevent a recurrence of all these problems. These might only consist of a warning not to aggravate the condition by performing any unusually strong activity. If the patient's occupation is the cause of tenovaginitis, however, it may be necessary to attempt to change or alter the work so that it is less repetitive. Splinting can sometimes give support so that less stress is put on the tendons.

## REFERENCES

Birch R, Grant C 1986 Periphal Nerve Injuries—Clinical. In: Downie P A (ed) Cash's Textbook of Neurology for Physiotherapists. Faber and Faber, London

Bunnell S T 1970 Surgery of the hand, 5th edn. Blackwell, Oxford

Dellon A L 1984 Touch sensibility in the hand. Journal of Hand Surgery 9B: 1

Frampton V M 1986 Problems in managing reconstructive surgery for brachial plexus lesions contrasted with peripheral nerve lesions. Journal of Hand Surgery 11B(1)

Harrison S H, Morris A 1975 Dupuytren's Contracture: the dorsal transposition flap. The Hand 7: 2

Jones S 1979 Investigation of brachial plexus traction lesions by peripheral and spinal somatosensory evoked potentials. Journal of Neurology, Neurosurgery & Psychiatry

Kleinert H E, Kutz J E, Atasoy E, Stormo A 1973 Primary repair of flexor tendons. Orthopaedic Clinics of North America 4(4)

Kleinert H E, Leitch I, Smith D J, Lubbers L M 1982 In:

Strickland & Steichen (ed) Difficult problems in hand surgery. Mosby, London

McCallum P, Hueston J T 1962 The pathology of Dupuytren's contracture. The Australian and New Zealand Journal of Surgery 31: 241–253

McCash C R 1964 The open palm technique in Dupuytren's contracture. British Journal of Plastic Surgery 17: 271

McGrouther D A, Ahmed M R 1981 Flexor tendon excursions in 'No-Man's Land'. The Hand 13: 129–141

Roberts M, Rutherford J H, Harris D 1982 The effect of ultrasound on flexor tendon repairs in the rabbit. The Hand 14: 1

Savage R 1985 In vitro studies of a new method of flexor repair. Journal of Hand Surgery 10B: 2

Semple C 1979 The primary management of hand injuries. Pitman, London

Slattery P G, McGrouther D A 1984 A modified Kleinert

controlled mobilisation splint following flexor tendon repair. Journal of Hand Surgery 9B: 2

Smith P J, Boardman S 1986 Primary repair of flexor tendon injuries in 'No-Man's Land'. Physiotherapy 72: 2

Verdan C L 1960 Primary repair of flexor tendons. Journal of Bone & Joint Surgery 42A: 647–657

Wilson D M 1983 Tenosynovitis, tendonvaginitis and trigger finger. Physiotherapy 69: 10

Wynn Parry C B 1981 Rehabilitation of the hand. Butterworths, London

Wynn Parry C B 1984 Symposium on Sensation. Journal of Hand Surgery 9B(1)

Wynn Parry C B, Salter M 1976 Sensory re-education after median nerve lesions. The Hand 8: 250–256

## FURTHER READING

Caillet R 1982 Hand pain and impairment. Davis, Philadelphia

Lister G 1984 The hand: diagnosis and indications, 2nd edn. Churchill Livingstone, Edinburgh

Mannerfelt L 1966 Studies on the hand in ulnar nerve paralysis. Acta Orthopaedica Scandinavia, Suppl 87. Munksgaard, Copenhagen

Omer G E, Spinner M 1980 Management of peripheral nerve lesions. Saunders, London

Salter M I 1986 Peripheral nerve injuries—physiotherapy. In Downie P A (ed) Cash's textbook of neurology for physiotherapists. Faber and Faber, London

# 5

# The burnt hand
*A.T. Davis*

The hand is particularly at risk from burn injury because of its exposed position and functional importance. We use it as a tool at work, and it frequently comes into contact with hot objects and liquids. In cases of fire the hand is instinctively used to put out flames and to protect the face. It is not surprising, therefore, that approximately 40% of all burn injuries involve the hand. However, the burnt hand is often only a part of a more extensive injury. Since the first priority in treatment is always to save life, the care of the hand may initially be of secondary importance but it must not be neglected in the subsequent overall management of the patient.

Although the area of the hand affected by the burn may be small it is still of great importance. Thermal injury and the resultant scarring and contracture can greatly affect hand function. Correct early management and treatment are therefore essential if maximum mobility and function of hand are to be maintained.

## CLASSIFICATION

Burns may be classified into three groups according to their cause as follows:
1. Thermal
   a. Flash and flame
   b. Contact with hot liquids or objects
   c. Steam
2. Electrical
3. Chemical.
Burns due to thermal agents are the most common.

## CHARACTERISTIC PATTERNS

Burns of the hand may show characteristic patterns, according to their cause.

### Flash burn

This is a common injury because of the exposed position of the hand at work and when it is protecting the face. The dorsum is the main area involved.

### Flame burn

In situations resulting in flame injury the hand is normally held clenched or against the face as protection. The dorsum is therefore the area most often involved. If the hand is used in an attempt to extinguish the flames, the palm and finger tips may be more severely affected. This type of burn is usually deep and other areas of the body are often involved.

### Contact burn

This results from grasping a hot object and may cause devastating damage to tissues in the fingers and palm (Fig. 5.1). In industrial accidents the dorsum may also be involved, for example when the hand is caught in a hot press.

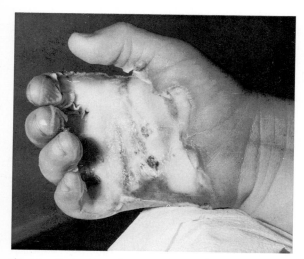

**Fig. 5.1** Contact burn from grasping a radiator bar fire.

### Electrical burn

In these cases the damage is due to the passage of an electric current causing a heating effect in the tissues. The amount of damage depends on the resistance of the skin and underlying tissues, on the duration of the current and on the presence of metal contacts (e.g. rings, bracelets etc.). There will always be an entrance and exit burn with hidden tissue damage between the two. The electrical burns seen most often are those involving the domestic 240 volt alternating current. Much more serious damage will be seen in injuries caused by direct current such as contact with electric railway lines or power cables.

### Chemical burn

These burns will be deep because the chemicals may penetrate into the tissues and have a prolonged effect.

## DEPTH OF BURN

The depth of tissue destruction will depend on many factors including the causative agent, the temperature to which the tissues are exposed and the duration of exposure. Tissue destruction can occur at temperatures as low as 45°C (a very hot bath), provided contact is maintained for long enough. Further tissue destruction can occur as a result of infection.

The depth of the burn will determine whether the wound will heal spontaneously or will require grafting. Any surviving islands of epidermis around the hair follicles, sebaceous and sweat glands in the burn area will provide new epidermal cells. In time these will spread to resurface and heal the burn wound.

Burns are described as being either superficial, partial or full thickness. Many burns are of mixed depth (see Fig. 5.2).

### Superficial

These burns are confined to the epidermis and superficial dermis. They result in a wet burn with many blisters, characterised by a red base. The wound is painful but heals quickly in 7–10 days.

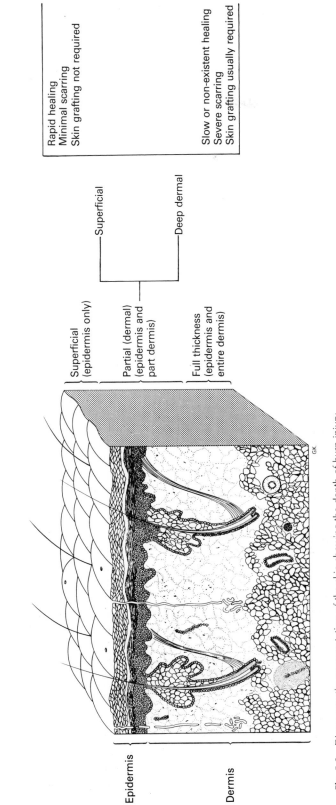

**Fig. 5.2** Diagrammatic representation of the skin showing the depth of burn injury.

Epidermis

Dermis

Superficial (epidermis only)

Partial (dermal) (epidermis and part dermis)

Full thickness (epidermis and entire dermis)

Superficial

Deep dermal

Rapid healing
Minimal scarring
Skin grafting not required

Slow or non-existent healing
Severe scarring
Skin grafting usually required

GK

## Partial

In partial thickness burns the damage extends more deeply into the dermis. There are a few blisters, which have a white base, and the wound may be insensitive to pin prick. The depth may be converted to a full thickness injury if the wound becomes infected. These burns should heal in 2–4 weeks, depending on how many undamaged epidermal cells survive to provide a source of new epidermis. However, hypertrophic scarring and contracture are common with the deeper partial thickness burns (deep dermal burns), which will take more than 18 days to heal.

## Full thickness

These burns destroy the full thickness of the skin and are characterised by a charred or white waxy appearance with visible thrombosed veins and no blisters. They are insensitive to pin prick. Spontaneous healing cannot occur as all the epidermal skin elements are destroyed. Healing can therefore only occur from the edges, and in the larger burns skin grafting will be necessary.

## PATHOLOGY OF THE WHOLE BURN INJURY

Following a burn injury the heat destroys the skin to a greater or lesser extent and tissue necrosis occurs. This area of necrosis is surrounded by a layer of tissue which, although severely affected by heat, is still viable. Pathological changes occur in these heat-affected tissues.

The main changes are dilation of the capillaries and an increase in capillary permeability, resulting in the passage of plasma into the extracellular spaces. This causes the blisters, if the skin surface is intact, exudate if the skin surface is broken, and gross oedema of the surrounding tissue spaces.

The loss of plasma occurs rapidly in the first few hours following the burn. It then gradually diminishes over the next two days as the capillaries recover, and the fluid within the tissue spaces is absorbed back into the circulation. If the burn area is large this fluid loss causes a decrease of circulating blood volume and may result in hypovolaemic shock with the eventual death of the patient if left untreated.

## SIZE OF BURN

The amount of plasma lost depends on the size of the burned surface so it is essential that the extent of the burn is estimated by the doctor at the onset of treatment.

The area of burn injury can be approximately estimated by Wallace's 'Rule of nines'. The head and neck is equal to 9% of the total body surface area, each upper limb 9%, each lower limb 18%, the front of the trunk 18%, the back 18% and the perineum is equivalent to the remaining 1%. The surface area covered by the patient's hand approximates to 1%. The Lund and Browder charts are a much more accurate and detailed method of measuring the size of burn injuries. For example, they take into account the disproportionate size of the developing child's head in relation to his body. When assessing the size of burn, by whichever method, the erythema around the burn is not included as part of the percentage of the area of body surface burnt.

Any burn greater than 10% of body surface area in a child, or 15% in an adult, will require immediate and urgent replacement of body fluid by means of an intravenous drip to prevent hypovolaemic shock. Many different replacement fluids are used and there are different formulae for estimating the volume of fluid required and rate of replacement, each Burns Unit favouring its own regime. In all instances, the fluid used acts as a plasma expander to maintain circulating blood volume.

In burns of less than 10% or 15% of body surface area, as in a burn involving the hand, the patient is able to compensate for the fluid loss by constriction of blood vessels in the gut and skin and by the redistribution of fluid from undamaged extracellular spaces. Thirst results, with more liquids being taken orally.

## MANAGEMENT OF THE BURN WOUND

Immediate treatment of any burn consists of maintenance of the airway, assessment of the wound, analgesia, tetanus prophylaxis and fluid replacement as indicated. From the start the wound should be treated aseptically as far as possible, since immediately following burn injury the wound surface is sterile as the heat will have destroyed the skin flora and bacteria.

Treatment of the burnt hand has two main aims:
1. To ensure rapid healing of the burn wound by an appropriate method.
2. Restoration of mobility and function as soon as possible.

Infection must be kept to a minimum, as this not only delays healing but also deepens burn injury.

Any delay in healing lengthens the potential period of impaired function and immobility, and increases the amount of scarring, fibrosis and contracture due to the excessive formation of granulation tissue. Granulation tissue is formed as part of the body's natural healing process. It is rich in capillaries (and therefore red in colour) and due to the large number of myofibrils amongst the collagen, it tends to contract, predisposing to deformities. Some healthy granulation tissue may be essential for wound healing and skin grafting, but if possible skin cover should be achieved before the development of excess granulation tissue, approximately 3–4 weeks post-burn.

Following evaluation and assessment of the burnt hand a plan of treatment is determined by the surgeon, bearing in mind that the sooner the hand is healed the better will be the long-term results. The preservation of function is more important than the appearance. A hand that works is preferable to a hand that may look good but functions poorly.

**Superficial and partial thickness burns**

Superficial and partial thickness burns of the hand, especially if part of a more extensive burn injury, are treated conservatively. Healing should occur within approximately two to three weeks by the growth of epidermis from the surviving islands of epidermis.

Following cleansing and deroofing of the larger blisters, the burns are covered with an antibacterial cream (for example silver sulphadiazine), and placed within a polythene bag, sealed at the wrist or forearm with gauze and a bandage (Fig. 5.3). This bag is changed daily, or more frequently in the first few days as exudate collects in the bag. Each dressing change is preceded by a gentle wash

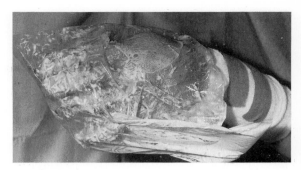

**Fig. 5.3** Hand bag with antibacterial cream, bandaged at the wrist.

and cleansing of the burn surface. The 'hand-bag' method of treatment is preferred by doctor, patient and therapist for it allows the wound to be viewed through the bag, is pain-free (except during dressing changes when the patient may complain of a stinging sensation) and permits free movement and exercise.

If healing does not occur within two to three weeks, surgery will be required, although given time, the wound would eventually heal itself. However, this application of skin grafts speeds up the healing process, encourages the restoration of function and decreases the degree of scarring and fibrosis.

*Surgical management*

Thin split skin grafts are used as these adhere or 'take' more rapidly, so allowing earlier postoperative mobilisation. Being thin they have a greater tendency to contract later, unless preventative measures are taken.

A bulky dressing is applied following grafting and left intact until the first dressing is performed at about five days. Thereafter non-bulky dressings, allowing freedom of movement, are applied until the grafts are stable and well healed (Fig. 5.4). Once the burn has healed, light dressings may be applied to protect the new thin epithelium which is easily damaged.

Localised deeper partial thickness burns, i.e. deep dermal burns of the hand, may be treated by early surgery involving 'tangential excision' and skin grafting at four to five days post-burn. The burn wound is shaved layer by layer until all

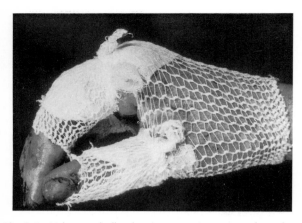

**Fig. 5.4** Light, non-bulky dressings covering new grafts and protecting thin epithelium.

necrotic tissue is removed, providing a healthy surface upon which thin skin grafts are applied. The take of grafts is usually excellent, allowing early and rapid rehabilitation, and there is minimal hypertrophic scarring or loss of function (Figs. 5.5, 5.6 & 5.7).

**Full thickness burns**

Surgery is inevitable following a full thickness burn injury to the hand, as all the epidermal elements in the burn wound have been destroyed. The hand burn may be associated with other burns and the surgeon's ideal choice and timing of treatment is then immediately limited by more urgent problems in other regions.

*Surgical management*

Severe constricting oedema may occur following deep circumferential burns of the upper limb and hand. If left untreated this may result in vascular compression and eventually ischaemic necrosis

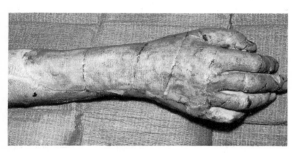

**Fig. 5.5**

**Figs. 5.5, 5.6, 5.7** Tangential excision showing good take of grafts and excellent functional and cosmetic result.

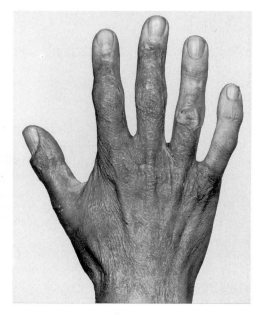

**Fig. 5.6**

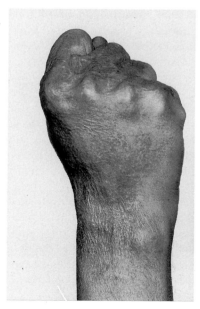

**Fig. 5.7**

distal to the constriction. Release incisions along the entire length of the constriction, through the necrosed tissues, allows expansion and the restoration of the circulation. An anaesthetic is not required.

If the patient's condition permits, early excision is preferred, to remove all necrotic tissue so that a clean surgical wound is ensured. This decreases the risk of infection. Prior to this surgery, the hand will be treated either in closed dressings or in a hand bag. Surgery may have to be delayed if the hand burn is part of a more extensive and serious injury.

Following excision of the deep burns to the extensor surface of the hand, skin grafts are applied but no take of graft is to be expected over exposed tendon or bone. After about 2–3 weeks a healthy layer of granulation tissue will form over these small areas which can then be covered with skin grafts. This may result in some residual stiffness due to delayed healing and to the contractile bed upon which the skin grafts were placed.

Extensive exposure of extensor tendons can be covered with a flap, usually from the groin, for 10–14 days. The flap is then removed leaving a small amount of vascular fat from beneath the flap to cover the exposed tendons and bones. Skin grafts can be applied to cover this new, healthy and viable bed. Restoration of mobility will be slow as the hand will be relatively immobile beneath the flap, and at least a week must be allowed following grafting before commencing exercises. Vigorous physiotherapy will then be required. Results are usually slow and can be less than ideal. Covering with a flap may be impossible in an extensive injury and healing of exposed tendons may have to await the growth of granulation tissue and delayed grafting.

Deep injuries to the palmar surface usually result from contact burns and often occur in isolation. In adults early excision and cover with a flap, usually from the groin, is the best course of treatment. Following separation and inset of the flap at 2–3 weeks, aggressive physiotherapy is commenced to restore maximum mobility and function (Fig. 5.8, 5.9 & 5.10). Further surgery to thin the flap may be required at a later date.

In children these deep palmar contact burns are best treated in polythene bags; this encourages as much use of the hand as possible whilst healing

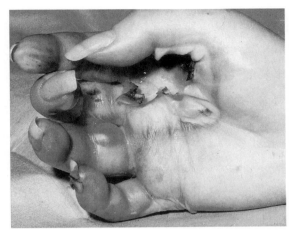

**Fig. 5.8**

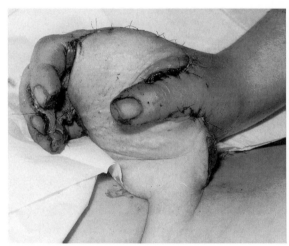

**Fig. 5.9**

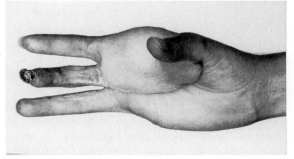

**Fig. 5.10**

**Figs. 5.8, 5.9, 5.10** Contact burn inset into a groin flap. Good functional result, with amputation of non-viable little finger.

occurs. Healing will be slow, usually taking about 4–6 weeks. Elective re-surfacing with thick grafts once healing is complete will give better results than early grafting. Further surgery and grafting is often needed as the hand grows, especially during adolescence.

Small localised deep burns, for example following an electrical burn of the fingers, are best covered with local flaps, but limited movement is still frequently the end result (Fig. 5.11). If the injury is so deep that there is permanent damage to the neuro-vascular bundles, even worse results can be expected.

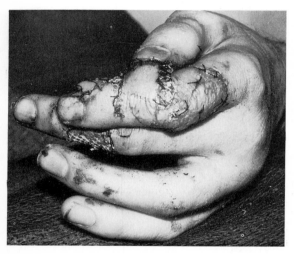

**Fig. 5.11** Local flaps covering small deep burns to finger tips and thumb.

Following deep burns of the fingers, joint surfaces may be exposed. If a single joint is exposed, it is immobilised until the skin heals. Once healing has occurred, the joint can be gently mobilised and return of function encouraged. Multiple open joints, however, pose a major problem. Unless early healing over exposed joints can be achieved, internal fixation with pins should be avoided due to the risk of infection. Positioning can be provided either by splints or by syndactylysing adjacent fingers and dividing them at a later stage, thus utilising the stability offered by neighbouring fingers. Amputation of a non-viable part of the hand may be indicated.

## STRUCTURAL CHANGES FOLLOWING BURN INJURY

Following burn injury the anatomy and thus function of the hand can be severely affected due to the soft tissue loss and damage. The fragility and adherence of skin grafts to the underlying tissues and their tendency to contract can all pose problems in the rehabilitation of the burnt hand.

The skin in the palm of the hand is thick and cornified and protects the underlying structures. Because of this, the palm is usually spared serious injury and the burn heals spontaneously. In the deeper devastating burn, the thick skin no longer offers sufficient protection to the deeper structures so that these may also be damaged.

The dorsal skin, however, is thin, elastic and very mobile, enabling it to stretch as the joints flex. It is easily damaged by thermal injury, often requiring skin grafting. Following injury there is frequently reduction of the normal elasticity and mobility, and movements become restricted.

The long flexors of the fingers are buried deep to the palmar fascia. Only a devastating injury will involve these tendons and such an injury inevitably compromises the whole function of the hand.

The long extensor tendons lie just beneath the thin dorsal skin and are thus easily damaged. If the

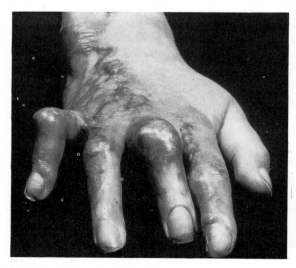

**Fig. 5.12** Boutonnière deformities.

central slip of the extensor expansion over the proximal interphalangeal joint is destroyed, the lateral bands may slip volarwards, becoming flexors of the joint and thus causing the classic boutonnière deformity (Fig. 5.12). Even if the central slip is intact following injury, it may subsequently be damaged by the poor positioning of joints, by oedema or by infection.

The mobile bony arches of the hand, so important for hand function, can all become immobile, flattened and even reversed following burn injury. A flat archless hand is incapable of cupping, gripping and opposing thumb to finger tip.

The thumb, by virtue of its anatomy and loose web skin, has great freedom of movement. Following burn injury the web may quickly tighten and contract, pulling the thumb flat against the index finger. In this position the excursion of the thumb will be limited and thumb to finger tip opposition will become impossible. Hand function will be severely affected.

## LATER RECONSTRUCTIVE SURGERY

Despite the efforts of all concerned, some burnt hands heal with joint impairment and contractures. Further surgery may then be indicated to improve function.

Frequently the thumb web will need releasing and the finger webs deepening by the use of local flaps or full thickness skin grafts. Contractures of the flexor aspects of the fingers, due to skin shortage, are corrected by the release of the contracture and insertion of a thick skin graft into the resultant defect. Thin skin grafts on the dorsum of the hand, if adherent to the underlying structures, will often result in limited flexion of the metacarpophalangeal joints. These grafts may be excised and replaced by thicker or larger skin grafts.

Very little can be achieved surgically to improve tendon function, especially of the extensor tendons, but tenolysis or manipulation of the joint under anaesthesia may be considered. A severely deformed stiff digit that impedes function may be fused into a more functional position or amputated in order to improve use and function in the rest of the hand.

## PSYCHOLOGICAL PROBLEMS FOLLOWING BURN INJURY

It is important to appreciate the patient's response to burn injury, especially a burn involving the hand. The hand is such a functional tool that if damaged by burn injury, it can render that patient dependent on others. There are three stages in the patient's response to injury; numbing shock, growing awareness and finally acceptance. These three stages can be recognised even in those who have only suffered burns of the hands. All affect the patient's behaviour reactions and for this reason care and understanding is needed when treating these patients.

Initially, there is a stage of acute mental shock at the loss of health, independence and the anticipation of permanent disfigurement and incapacity. Few patients have any comparable experience of such an injury. Their fears and anxieties may be accentuated by the isolation necessary in early burn management. The response of the burnt patient to his acute injuries may be observed either as withdrawal into personal isolation, with total passive submission and dependence, or as protest and complaint, characterised by speech obscenities, violence and non co-operation.

Gradually the patient will pass through this shock phase into the second stage. In this period he experiences a growing awareness of the injury sustained and all that it entails. He may ask himself what happened and why; he may attempt to attach blame to others and may long 'to put back the clock'. Depression is inevitable but should never become a permanent feature. It is a natural response to all serious injury, to functional disabilities, to the prospect of a series of dressings and surgical procedures, to the feeling of uselessness and to the cosmetic blemishes that may be developing.

Rehabilitation and the recovery of independence and self-respect cannot be achieved until the patient finally accepts what has occurred. In this phase, complete frankness is essential to assist the patient in coming to terms with the injury. The treatment plans and procedures involved, what to expect and what can be achieved, the long-term prospects of physical recovery, disfigurement and scarring, and the return to the family and to the job are all carefully and truthfully explained and discussed with the patient.

Not all patients pass smoothly from one stage to the next. Some will demonstrate true psychiatric disturbances, but this will depend primarily on the pre-burn personality.

For the physiotherapist it is important to try and gain the patient's co-operation and maximum effort throughout all stages of treatment. This can at times be difficult to achieve and will depend on the patient's own behavioural response to injury. Much time, patience and understanding is needed and each stage of treatment must be fully explained to the patient. The physiotherapist's approach and attitude is all important. It must be sympathetic yet firm in order to achieve the necessary goals.

## PHYSIOTHERAPY FOR THE BURNT HAND

Physiotherapy treatment can be divided into two stages: the early or acute stage, in which the recently burnt hand is treated, and the later healed or post-surgery stage, where the main emphasis is on rehabilitation. In reality this is not a clear-cut division, as one stage progresses into the other.

Physiotherapy is started as soon as possible following injury. Success in treating the burnt patient depends on the co-operation of the whole Burns Unit team including surgeon, nurse, physiotherapist, occupational therapist, medical social worker, family doctor and disablement resettlement officer, together with the patient and his family.

The main aims of treatment are to:
1. Reduce oedema
2. Maintain joint range
3. Minimise the formation of contractures and deformity
4. Restore maximum function possible.

### Acute stage

#### Treatment of oedema

Initially pain and oedema are the main obstacles in regaining full range of movement. Following injury the burnt hand will quickly assume a poor position, with developing contracture and deformity. In this position the wrist becomes flexed and radially deviated with extension or hyperextension

of the metacarpophalangeal (MCP) joints, flexion of the interphalangeal (IP) joints and adduction of the thumb. This is the characteristic claw hand deformity. (Fig. 5.13).

In the acute burn this position is usually due to oedema. (Fig. 5.14). If this oedema is not dispersed early, the hand will remain in the clawed position and normal movement patterns will gradually become more difficult. As the persistent oedema organises and fibrosis occurs, the small gliding movements between the bones will diminish, the arches will flatten, the soft tissues will become bound together and gradually the hand will become fixed. Therefore, from the first moment possible the burnt hand must be elevated to keep the oedema to a minimum and to assist its dispersal by gravity. The arm can be elevated using pillows or foam and wire support, or suspended in a sling or roller towel from a drip-stand. If it is a minor hand burn being treated on an out-patient basis, it

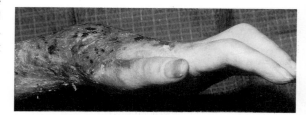

**Fig. 5.13** Clawed hand deformity.

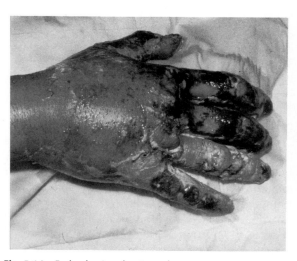

**Fig. 5.14** Early clawing due to oedema.

can be elevated in an arm sling. Small range pumping exercises performed in elevation will also assist the absorption of oedema by increasing the venous return.

*Splinting*

If the patient is unwilling or unable to maintain his hand in the position of anti-contracture, a paddle splint can be applied over the hand bag to correct the clawed position. (Fig. 5.15). In this corrected position the wrist should be splinted in extension with 90° flexion at the MCP joints together with full extension of the IP joints, with the thumb abducted and extended to maintain the first web space. The splint can be made from thermoplastic materials or from plaster of Paris. It can be moulded directly over the hand bag or dressing. Initially, oedema may prevent the optimum position from being achieved, but as the oedema subsides during the first few days, so the splint should be adjusted or remade to correct the position.

Careful supervision is needed as prolonged splinting must be avoided. As soon as the pain and oedema allow more movement and the patient becomes more co-operative, the splint can be removed for periods during the day to allow for exercises and activities of daily living (feeding, drinking etc.). In time the splint need only be worn at night, provided that the patient is freely using his hand during the day and is able to maintain MCP joint flexion and IP joint extension.

In the full thickness burn of the dorsum, care must be taken to protect any exposed extensor tendons. The paddle splint may be worn continuously, only being removed for careful exercise under the supervision of the physiotherapist.

Individually designed splints may also be needed during the acute phase, for example a thumb web splint to maintain thumb abduction or a small gutter splint to protect a single exposed extensor tendon.

*Exercise*

Exercises are started from the day of injury and a full range of movement is the ultimate goal. If the patient is reluctant to exercise, some gentle manual assistance should be given to channel the patient's effort and to help him to achieve all that he is physically capable of doing. Any passive movements must be performed with care as they can cause further damage, oedema and haemorrhage resulting in further restriction of joint range. Active and assisted active exercises are preferable as they help maintain muscle strength and normal movement patterns.

As the oedema subsides the joint range will increase. The hand bag allows complete freedom of movement. Activities of daily living are also encouraged. In this way exercise is translated into function. (Fig. 5.16). Some patients need constant encouragement and persuasion to move and use their hands prior to healing. It is too late to wait until healing has occurred before starting exercises, as fibrosis and stiffness will have begun to limit hand use and function.

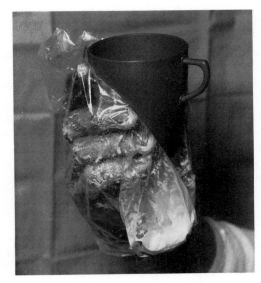

**Fig. 5.16** Hand bag allowing gripping and complete freedom of movement.

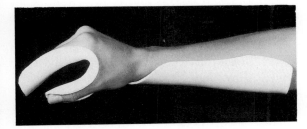

**Fig. 5.15** Paddle splint.

The following exercises are performed, and the physiotherapist will work with the patient several times a day until full range of movement, or the best range of movement possible is achieved.
1. Full finger extension, abduction and adduction
2. Full wrist and thumb movements
3. Thumb to finger tip opposition
4. MCP joint flexion with IP joint extension
5. IP joint flexion with MCP joint extension.

In deep dermal and full thickness burns, fist-making and passive proximal IP joint flexion are not allowed as they may jeopardise the extensor tendon.

If the burn involves the whole upper limb, it too must be correctly positioned and exercised. The limb is elevated, positioned and exercised to maintain at least 90° abduction at the shoulder and full elbow extension.

Even if the burn only involves the hand, the rest of the upper limb must be kept mobile. General arm exercises are performed as a stiff shoulder or elbow will affect hand function in the future. Pronation and supination must not be neglected.

This regime of correct positioning, splinting and exercise is continued until healing has occurred, or skin grafts are applied. Following grafting the hand is immobilised and splinted in the correct position and left elevated until the first dressing. This is normally on the fifth day but may be performed earlier if required, because of sudden pain and discomfort, or obvious oozing or bleeding. A light non-bulky dressing is then applied and changed on alternate days for as long as is necessary. The donor site dressing is left intact for 10 days, by which time it should have nearly healed.

If the hand has been covered with a flap, the mobility of the 'free' joints should be maintained. Modified movements of the shoulder, elbow and wrist are also encouraged. The position of the hand is maintained with strapping and foam pads to prevent a kink or tension in the flap which could jeopardise its viability.

## Post-healing rehabilitation

Following healing or grafting the new skin and grafts are thin and fragile and blister easily. Careful handling is therefore required, but mobility

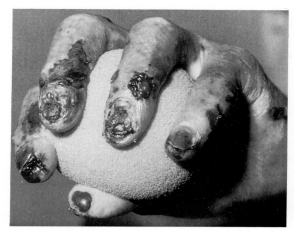

**Fig. 5.17** Rehabilitation must continue regardless of blisters and nail damage.

and exercise must nevertheless be maintained (Fig. 5.17). Gentle exercise of the grafted areas is commenced once the grafts are stable, usually at 5–7 days. It is essential to restore range of movement, although wounds may still be unhealed in places. General mobility exercises are performed and the use of hand in activities of daily living is encouraged. If limited movement is present, formal exercises are given to regain the range. Exercising in water or silicone oil can be beneficial and emphasis on MCP joint flexion, IP joint flexion and extension and thumb abduction and opposition is essential at this stage.

As the grafts stabilise they are gently creamed in order to keep them greasy and supple. The patient is instructed to do this as often as is necessary to prevent dry scaling or cracking, using a bland soft cream. Should blisters occur, a light dressing or zinc oxide tape is applied over the open area until dry and healed.

As the skin matures, so massaging can become deeper to soften fibrosis and to loosen any contracted soft tissue. Ultrasound to isolated tight areas can be effective, but usually the fibrosis is too extensive. Passive stretches can be given to restore limited movement, but these must be gentle, slow and sustained in order to avoid traumatising the joints and increasing the fibrosis. Heat treatment, hot water and wax baths must be avoided, as the new skin is exceedingly thin and may be insensitive to temperature.

Following massage and stretching, exercises and activities are performed to mobilise and strengthen the hand further. Much imagination on the part of the physiotherapist is necessary to prevent repetition. Free active exercise, manipulation of objects, squeezing a foam ball, weight and pulley exercises to strengthen the upper limb and grip, proprioceptive neuromuscular facilitation techniques and weight-bearing exercises through the hand, are some of the methods available to achieve hand mobility and function.

The paddle splint may still be being worn at night, the patient resting his hand with wrist in extension, MCP joints in flexion and IP joints in extension. The splint must be well padded and applied carefully so as to prevent skin breakdown.

The potential for contractures to develop can last for many months, so exercising to stretch the new skin and grafts should continue well after healing has occurred. The patient should be made aware of how important this is. He may have been discharged from hospital, in which case regular out-patient appointments must be organised, if necessary, at a local hospital when travelling distance to the Burns Unit is too great. Regular follow-up appointments should be arranged by the Burns Unit, and communication between the Unit and the local physiotherapy department should be frequent and accurate.

The role of the physiotherapist at this stage is particularly important, for the patient often goes home with high expectations only to find that everything is much more difficult or even impossible. At each out-patient attendance, problems can be discussed and, hopefully, resolved; morale and self-confidence can be boosted; encouragement and support given. The physiotherapist can act as a good listener and is a useful link between the patient and the surgeon, alerting the latter to troublesome problems, developing contractures and functional limitations.

The rehabilitation following major surgery which may include flap repair, fusion of joints or amputation, will be individualised to each patient's needs. The same goals apply: achieving maximum mobility, strength and function. Careful assessment is essential to evaluate the hand's potential and capabilities.

## OCCUPATIONAL THERAPY

The occupational therapy department has much to offer for the rehabilitation of the burnt hand. Treatment available includes assisting the patient with activities of daily living and function, producing necessary adaptations, encouraging activities, games and at a later stage heavier workshop activities, and providing assistance with job assessment and retraining if necessary. Some OT departments are responsible for the fabrication of splints and the application of pressure garments.

### Pressure garments

Following healing, there is a long phase of scar maturation, during which time the scar remains active and will readily shorten and contract. This is a most important phase in patient management as this constant threat of contracture must be opposed by exercise, stretching, splinting and by the use of pressure garments.

Hypertrophic scarring develops in 70–80% of all burn scars, especially the deep dermal burns allowed to heal spontaneously, between grafted areas and sometimes in the grafts themselves, for it is the bed which becomes hypertrophic. Frequently the patient may be discharged with a satisfactory appearance and function, but within three to four weeks these scars begin to hypertrophy. They become red, itchy, raised, thick and gnarled. They not only look unsightly but will result in limited joint mobility and contractures (Fig. 5.18).

Once the skin on the burnt hand has healed, the patient should be fitted with a pressure glove. These gloves, which permit full hand activity, will decrease hypertrophic scarring and help maintain scar elasticity, thereby promoting joint mobility.

The pressure glove may be ready-made, or made to measure from either Lycra or Tubigrip (Figs. 5.19 & 5.20). The patient is encouraged to wear the glove day and night. All housework, activities, sport and employment are performed wearing the glove, and it is only removed for regular washing and skin care. During physiotherapy sessions the glove may be removed for a short time to allow specific stretching and mobilisation techniques; otherwise it is worn during all exercises and activities.

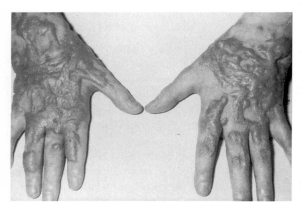

**Fig. 5.18** Hypertrophic scarring.

The hand should be completely healed before the glove is fitted, because the dorsal skin is so thin and delicate that the effect of pulling on the glove can easily enlarge small open areas, thus delaying healing. When applied the glove must fit correctly; the fingers should be pushed well into the glove so that good contact is made in the finger web spaces. The thumb must also be fully adjusted within the glove so that the thenar seam follows the thenar crease in the palm. If a pressure vest or sleeve is needed for applying pressure to the upper limb, there should be an overlap between glove and sleeve for full scar coverage.

Two pairs of gloves are provided and they are re-measured and re-fitted every three months. The regime of pressure can last for 12–18 months, after which time the scars will be fully mature and the risk of hypertrophy over. By the application of pressure the thick gnarled hypertrophic scarring is reduced, the itching is alleviated, a more elastic and pliable scar develops and less secondary surgery to relieve scar contracture is required.

## PHYSIOTHERAPY OF THE CONTRACTED BURNT HAND

Despite early elevation, splinting and exercise, and intensive rehabilitation and pressure therapy, some hands will heal with joint contractures and limitation of movement (Fig. 5.21). Contractures of the thumb web, hyperextension of the MCP joints and stiff IP joints exhibiting either flexion or extension contractures, are all too common. Intensive physiotherapy treatment may well alleviate

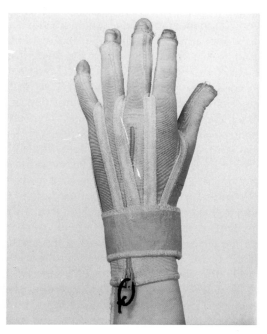

**Fig. 5.19** Made to measure Lycra glove with additional finger web separators.

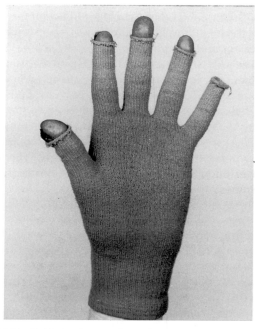

**Fig. 5.20** Tubigrip glove ready made.

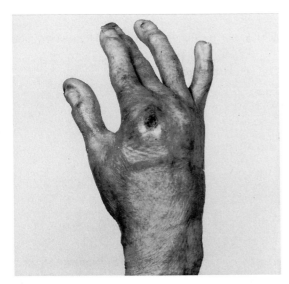

**Fig. 5.21**   Post-burnt hand showing joint contractures.

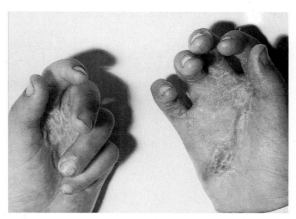

**Fig. 5.22**   Contractures in a child's hands due to skin shortages during growth (healed injury in Fig. 5.1).

some of the problems of the clawed hand, but surgery may also be indicated.

Frequent daily stretching, exercise and progressive splinting may reduce joint contractures. Should contractures of the thumb web occur, serial wedges can be made to increase abduction followed by a thermoplastic thenar splint to maintain maximum abduction. This should extend from the proximal IP joint of the index finger to the IP joint of the thumb, and be closely moulded to the thumb web contour.

Flexion contractures of the fingers are common, and following passive stretching and exercise a volar gutter splint may be applied. More elaborate lively traction splints can also be used, as can a well-padded dorsal paddle with finger loops, or a glove fitted with dorsal stiffening ribs. The little finger often poses special problems, for it quickly assumes a poor position of flexion and rotation.

Should tightening of the dorsal skin occur with limited MCP joint flexion, a flexion glove can be worn at night. A paddle splint with progressive flexion at the MCP joints can also be worn. With tightening of the dorsal skin, contractures of the web spaces often occur. Correct fitting of the pressure glove may be all that is required to resolve the problem, but additional finger separators may be worn in conjunction with the glove (Fig. 5.19). These can be made from either rolls

of foam or alternatively an extra Lycra garment can be fitted over the glove.

In the case of a child, the hand often becomes contracted, especially into flexion, as there is skin shortage as the hand grows (Fig. 5.22). Repeated assessment and careful splinting is essential. Unlike the adult, continuous splinting can be maintained for some time, as the child's hand quickly regains mobility and suppleness on removal of the splint.

In all instances, persistent contractures which limit hand function must be carefully reviewed and the possibilities of surgery can be considered and discussed with patient and surgeon.

Treating the burnt hand is a real challenge. With effective early management, correct positioning, splinting and exercise and prolonged after-care, mobility of the hand can be maintained and contractures reduced to a minimum so that the hand can remain a functional tool.

## ACKNOWLEDGEMENTS

I should like to thank Mr John Clarke FRCS Consultant Plastic Surgeon at Queen Mary's Hospital, Roehampton for his help and encouragement; the Department of Medical Photography, Queen Mary's Hospital, Roehampton, for their assistance in providing the photographic material; Mr G. Kotas BA MA AIMBI for his illustration and Mrs D. Browning and Mrs M. Lay for the many hours of typing.

## FURTHER READING

Cason J S 1981 Treatment of burns. Chapman & Hall, London

Davies D M 1985 Plastic and reconstructive surgery: burns. British Medical Journal 290: 989–993

Muir I F K, Barclay Th 1974 Burns and their treatment. Lloyd-Luke, London

Salisbury R E, Pruitt B A 1976 Burns of the upper extremity. Saunders, Philadelphia

# 6

# Occupational therapy and hand treatment

*H. Unsworth*

The treatment component in the occupational therapist's management of the injured hand usually includes the use of adapted activities. These activities are many and varied but of equal value are everyday tasks and games which offer simple repetitive movements appropriate to the stage of recovery reached. All activities, whether modified or not, are selected to suit the aims of treatment for the individual and as such form an important part of the team concept of rehabilitation.

The occupational therapist has three main areas in which treatment can be offered: by activities of daily living; by light workshop activities, e.g. early hand movements and basic re-education through adapted games, computers or light craftwork; and by heavy workshop activities, e.g. the use of hand tools, carpentry, medium to heavy engineering, welding etc. However, it is essential that the patient understands the aims of treatment and why he is performing a certain task, especially if it is a remedial game. Failure to do this will result in misinterpretation as the patient may feel that the session has been inappropriate and meaningless.

As in physiotherapy the treatment aims are divided into early, middle and late stages, but the best results are achieved by early intensive therapy from a combined hand team in which the physio and occupational therapists work closely together and have good liaison with the surgical team. In this way there is good co-operation between members of the rehabilitation team which is essential for clear goal setting and the understanding of the aims of treatment by all concerned.

## OCCUPATIONAL THERAPY FOLLOWING FLEXOR TENDON REPAIR

At three weeks post-surgery, following the removal of Kleinert traction and stitches, the patient may commence daily occupational therapy. However, the date at which therapy starts will vary according to the régime practised by individual units.

### EARLY STAGE

Upon initial referral at three weeks post repair, there are six main aims of treatment to be considered. These include assessment, the reduction of oedema, the increase of range, dexterity and hand-eye co-ordination, the care of skin and scars and the teaching of precautions.

### The accurate assessment of hand function

Weekly hand assessment should involve measurement of range of finger movement, sensation, hand volume, circulation, sweating and pain. In addition, note should be made of other relevant information such as pre-morbid disabilities, employment requirements and hobbies. Both active and passive range of movement should be measured, although the finger should *not* be pushed passively beyond the limitations of the extensibility of the flexor tendon until the six week stage has been reached. Measurement of hand power is similarly contra-indicated before six weeks post-repair.

Sensation for both light and deep touch should be assessed, plus an objective measurement such as the alteration of skin resistance.

### Reduction of oedema

Reduction should be achieved by the use of elevated activities and the necessary mobilisation of accessory joints, e.g. the elbow and shoulder, to improve circulation. Useful treatment activities to achieve this aim include all manner of wall-mounted games, e.g. large sized draughts or solitaire; some craftwork such as making a hanging basket by attaching macramé to a gantry; simple activities such as writing or playing games (e.g. hangman, noughts and crosses) on a blackboard;

and a group activity between two or more similar hand patients of keeping a balloon in the air. Numerous activities are suitable and although many are simple, it is essential that the patient gets variety in order to combat boredom at this stage when hand usage is so limited.

Care should be taken when choosing activities as arm movements must be active in order to achieve maximum benefit. Simply placing a game on a shelf may mean that the arm is static and results in minimal movement and a painful shoulder. Seating the patient to perform some elevated activities will eliminate compensatory movements such as standing on tiptoe and lateral trunk bending.

### To increase range of movement

The patient should be encouraged to mobilise all fingers actively, bearing in mind the limitations on the repaired tendons at this early stage. The wrist should also only be mobilised from the flexed to the mid or neutral position. Active and passive extension should be discouraged, as for the fingers, until the recommended six week stage has been reached.

Treatment activities may be the same as used for the reduction of oedema and should be supplemented by more dextrous tasks to encourage specific movements of the wrist and fingers. Once again these activities will vary depending upon the movement to be achieved. Essentially, any activity that does not offer resistance is acceptable and remedial games with or without adaptation can be of great benefit.

### To increase dexterity and hand-eye co-ordination

Skills of dexterity and hand-eye co-ordination are diminished following trauma and immobilisation. In addition, it is necessary to overcome the natural fear and reluctance to mobilise the hand and integrate it once more into the patient's concept of his body image. Encouragement should be given to the patient in order that he adopts a more normal arm posture and starts to re-use the hand in body language. It is therefore essential that time is spent in explaining basic anatomy and surgical procedure. This will have the dual purpose of calming the patient's apprehension about what has been done to his hand and also of reassuring him that the therapist is knowledgeable about both his condition and the limits to which he must work in therapy sessions. Useful activities to promote dexterity include manipulation of light small objects (such as pens, match sticks and playing cards), remedial games, type-setting, collating and sorting paperwork (for example course handouts and patient education leaflets), filing non-confidential cards and papers and light crafts such as painting and basketry. Writing skills may be practised where appropriate with writing patterns and doodling as a prerequisite to actual handwriting.

The electric typewriter and computer can also be useful. The latter may be used both as a word processor when writing is extremely difficult, illegible or slow, and also for computer games which require skills of speed and hand-eye co-ordination. Where ability permits some patients may compose simple new programs for others less able, e.g. patients with neurological or brain damage. This frequently has the desired effect of involving the patient in continuous and repetitive exercise whilst diverting his attention from his injury and relieving boredom by merit of a sufficiently interesting project.

### To give or reinforce appropriate skin and scar care

Attention should be paid to the removal of dead skin, hand cleanliness, the use of creams to improve skin quality, gentle massage to assist in maturation of the scar and the discouragement of tethering. All these procedures may be carried out by the physiotherapist, but again, awareness on the part of the occupational therapist may act as a useful reinforcement if the patient is to continue outside treatment hours. Similarly, this principle will also relate to the use of silicone oil for the promotion of skin healing and facilitation of mobilisation where it may be in use by either of the therapy departments. Where the circulation is poor the patient will generally complain of a cold hand. Wearing a glove will usually help to improve this problem, and it may be beneficial for him to wear a thermal vest in cold weather, thus keeping his trunk warm also. Commercial hand warmers

and special gloves may in some instances be of benefit. However, when a patient considers making his own version great care must be taken over the temperature of the heated object, especially when there is sensory loss.

### To teach precautions

It is vital to teach the patient appropriate precautions concerning care of the repaired tendons until six weeks post-surgery and also the care of the anaesthetic areas if there is nerve involvement. However, this teaching should be aimed at the reduction of fear and anxiety rather than the promotion of it and should therefore be tailored to the individual's needs rather than be given on a generalised basis. It is useful for this instruction to be linked to the patient's general education concerning his hand condition and surgery.

MIDDLE STAGE

When the patient is six weeks post-surgery, it is time to upgrade the treatment sessions in order to work for power, pinch grip and full finger extension. In addition, treatment should be aimed at the reduction of scar tissue and adhesions by the introduction of passive stretching. Activities in the light workshop can therefore be upgraded to offer some resistance, such as a solitaire game using spring clothes pegs or stool seating, and the patient will be introduced to the heavy workshop. Some hospitals may offer a comprehensive area as an adjunct to the occupational therapy department, comprising woodworking, engineering and electronic sections. These departments are staffed by carpenters and technicians as well as an occupational therapist. Other hospitals may have one area within the occupational therapy department, usually for woodworking with hand tools, staffed by an occupational therapist and occupational therapy technician.

In the heavy workshop, activities should be as carefully graded as in the light workshop. In addition to the stage of treatment reached, consideration must also be given to the patient's occupation and, wherever possible and appropriate, job simulation should be utilised to fulfil treatment aims.

Treatment activities in the heavy workshop should include the use of hand tools, e.g. sawing, hammering, chiselling and use of a screwdriver, hand sanding using a rectangular block to which the paper is tacked, grasping the block horizontally to encourage both finger flexion and grip strength, or pushing it along its vertical axis to promote finger and wrist extension. In larger workshops power tools can be used, for example power drills and electric sanders help to promote grip strength. Despite the use of power, these pieces of equipment still provide necessary resistance for grasp and movement.

At six weeks, it is quite likely that many patients will request permission to drive their car. Once the insurance company has been informed, there should be little problem. However, in cases where there is doubt, an assessment can be arranged at any British School of Motoring driving school.

Static splinting may now be used either as an adjunct to passive stretching in order to improve finger extension or to block certain joints whilst working for specific movements during occupational therapy activities. These splints can be made of thermoplastic materials to facilitate alteration as progress dictates. Small serial and blocking splints can be made for day use, whereas night splintage may also be offered in an effort to maintain the movement gained during the day.

Where there is also nerve damage, dynamic splinting may be used. In this instance, most occupational therapy departments either custom-make the devices (using a combination of spring-wire and springs and thermoplastic materials) or have access to a trained technician. In either instance, great care must be taken to ensure that the suitable amount of correction or assistance is achieved and that any resistance offered is appropriate to the progress that the patient has made. These splints may only be worn during treatment activities for a similar reason to the blocking splints, or they may be worn to prevent deformity and assist function as in ulnar nerve lesion correction.

At this stage it may be useful to use an unaffected finger to assist movement of the repaired one during activities. This can be done by the use of a 'Buddy' or by the making of a material loop to ensure that the two fingers work in unison.

## LATE STAGE

Gradually the work can be increased until the patient spends up to six hours a day doing heavy manual work. It should now be possible to conduct a realistic work assessment by the simulation of the patient's work environment. In this way not only is the assessor able to judge the patient's ability to conduct the job, but also to examine tolerance, fatigue levels and ability to return to work routine. It may be necessary for either the physio or occupational therapist to continue the passive stretching of the patient's hand at intervals throughout the working day if full passive finger extension has not been gained. However, the need to do this is reduced when the patient can assume this responsibility for himself, by exercise, splinting or by a combination of both.

Heavier tasks in the light workshop should now include such activities as printing using a hand press which may be adapted by either the addition of spring resistance or the use of a special handle, stool seating to promote skin toughening and gross grip, making plastic coated metal coathangers by the use of a hand jig, wrought iron work (forming the shapes by hand) or rivetting and using metal rivets. In the heavy workshop, activities should be similarly upgraded to promote general upper limb and hand strength plus toughening and redevelopment of hand callouses where relevant. Activities may then include cross-cut sawing, planing hardwood and the general use of heavier tools for longer periods of time. Once again, the activities offered will be dependent upon the facilities available in addition to the age and sex of the patient. Towards the end of his treatment session less time should be spent in physiotherapy and the light workshop and more in the heavy workshop, if it exists, where heavier activities can be offered.

## OTHER HAND CONDITIONS

Extensor tendon repairs will involve the same principals as for management of flexor tendons. Crush injuries, reflex sympathetic dystrophy and fractures will be managed according to the degree of hand trauma. Initial consideration by the occupational therapist is for activities that encourage a reduction of oedema and improvement in circulation by the encouragement of movements of the shoulder, elbow, wrist and fingers.

The therapist will be concerned with temperature of the limb, condition of the skin and severity of pain where it not only causes reluctance to move but also reinforces the protective posture, with the limb held closely to the body. In severe instances, where a patient is really reluctant to mobilise the arm, a limb balancer or OB Help Arm may be of assistance. This gravity-assist device, in which the weight of the arm is taken by slings and balanced by the use of lead weights, promotes smooth movements. At no time is the patient unable to control movement, although the occupational therapist is easily able to monitor and adjust the range offered. This equipment may be of particular use in reflex sympathetic dystrophy or shoulder-hand syndrome. The benefit of this sling system is that it offers equal support when the arm is in the extensor position, thus eliminating the problems of working with a flexed elbow and the subsequent constriction of circulation in the cubital fossa.

Other aims of treatment, such as increasing range of movement, power and assessment of any sensory deficit, will be the same as in the physiotherapy assessment and graded into early, middle and late stages.

## EXAMPLES OF ADAPTED ACTIVITIES

The following text gives specific examples of how the occupational therapist may adapt an activity in several different ways in order to fulfil the aims of treatment.

## THE SOLITAIRE GAME

The pocket sized version is very useful for dexterity and co-ordination, hand-eye co-ordination, opposition, sensory re-training, desensitisation and active flexion of the metacarpal and interphalangeal joints of the fingers. Further adaptations can be achieved by the positioning of the activity, as the following examples will show.

### Adaptation 1

Use of a wedge to encourage wrist flexion/extension:

*a. Wrist flexion*

(i) Place the game on the table, adjacent to the larger end of the wedge.
(ii) Rest the forearm along the wedge, so that the hand extends over the edge of it.
(iii) The patient therefore has to use the maximum wrist flexion to be able to reach the game (Fig. 6.1).

*b. Wrist extension*

(i) Rest the game at the topmost part of the wedge.
(ii) Rest the forearm on the remainder of the

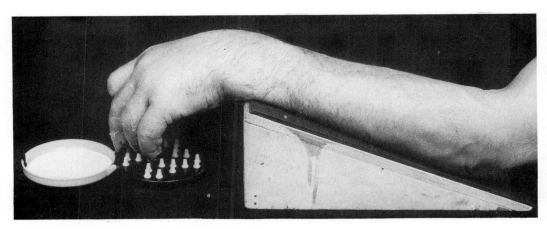

**Fig. 6.1** The use of a wedge helps to promote wrist flexion.

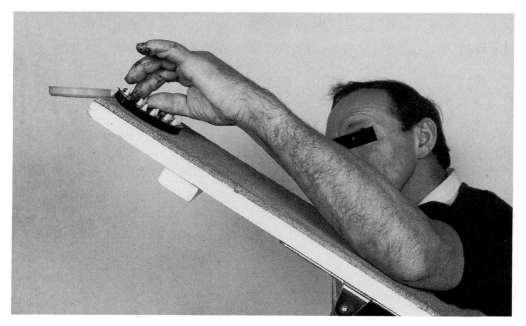

**Fig. 6.2** An elevated hand table is useful for a patient with marked oedema and minimal wrist extension.

wedge, whilst keeping the elbow on the table.
(If necessary make the patient hold his forearm down, by using his other hand.)
(iii) The patient therefore has to use maximum
wrist extension to play the game (Fig. 6.2).

### c. Pronation/Extension

To achieve these movements, the patient must
place his captured pieces into an adjacent container by supinating his forearm. Pronation will
occur when returning to the original position to
play the game.

### Adaptation 2

For metacarpophalangeal joint flexion, for combined finger opposition to improve the palmar
arch, and for sensory training or desensitisation,
the patient should remove the pieces from a box
via a hole cut out of the lid (Fig. 6.3).

### Adaptation 3

Tweezers and clothes pegs are very useful, especially when graded according to their spring resist-

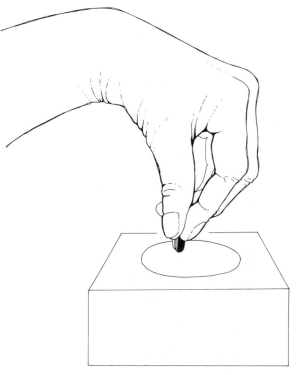

**Fig. 6.3** Removing the pieces through a hole cut in the box
assists wrist and MCP flexion and promotes finger dexterity.

ance. The movements achieved include opposition and static pinch grip, but the activity is equally effective for the encouragement of dexterity and coordination.

The tweezers and pegs should be graded according to their resistance and colour coded if necessary, and the tweezers padded with plastazote for increased passive extension.

## Adaptation 4

Large scale games, whether laid flat on a table, inclined or wall mounted on a graded height system, are useful for the reduction of oedema and the promotion of large active elbow and shoulder movements (Fig. 6.4). To discourage compensatory trunk side flexion it may be necessary to stabilise the pelvis by seating the patient.

When using extra large pieces, early opposition movements are also encouraged.

Pieces may be made out of 1 or 2 inch dowelling

rod (3–6 inches long), or any of the following shaped pieces (Fig. 6.5):

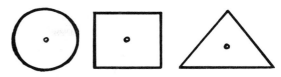

**Fig. 6.5** Different shapes may be used according to hand requirements.

## Further adaptations

(i) Increase the length of the dowelling rod pieces,
(ii) Weight the pieces with lead shot,
(iii) Make the game magnetic,
(iv) Use large rubber balls for pieces,
(v) Blindfold the patient to increase sensory stimulation,
(vi) To encourage internal and external rotation of the shoulder, place the container for the captured pieces in an appropriate position.

## THE SPAN GAME

There are many adaptations of this game, which when played in its entirety provides 132 moves. Simple modifications can be made to the size, bulk and weight of the pieces. Four such modifications are shown in Figure 6.6a. Limitations on the variation of these modifications are really only dependent upon the extent of the therapist's imagination, and access to a person who can make what is required.

The tallest model offers a good shoulder/hand range, useful in discouraging or dispersing oedema during early rehabilitation (Fig. 6.6b).

## NOUGHTS AND CROSSES

This simple game offers several alternatives, from encouraging large active arm movements in elevation by chalking on a blackboard, to extending the complexity of the game as in versions 1 and 2 (Figs. 6.7 and 6.8).

Further adaptations such as the use of weights and magnets or the attaching of pieces to velcro will add resistance. Once again, this should be

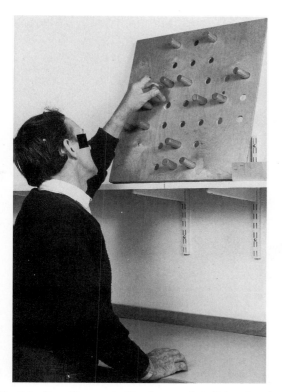

**Fig. 6.4** Dowelling used with a large scale solitaire placed in elevation.

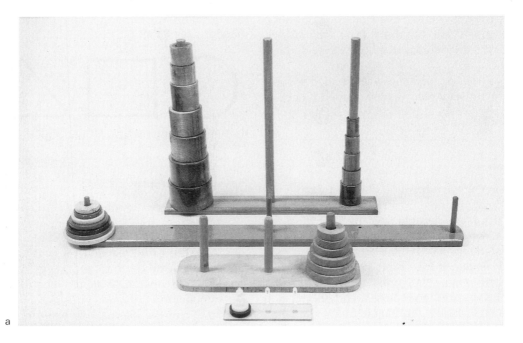

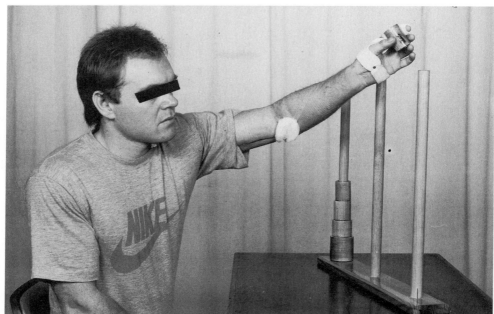

**Fig. 6.6(a & b)** Four adaptations for the span game. The tall model offers a good shoulder/hand range.

carefully graded if weights are involved. The weight of the arm can also be either assisted or resisted by the use of the limb balancer described earlier in this chapter.

COATHANGER 'TWISTERS'

Made from plastic coathanger wire and dowelling rod, these are essentially for wrist flexion/extension,

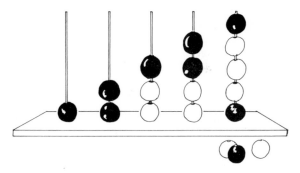

**Fig. 6.7** A variation of noughts and crosses using either wooden balls or tiny wooden beads.

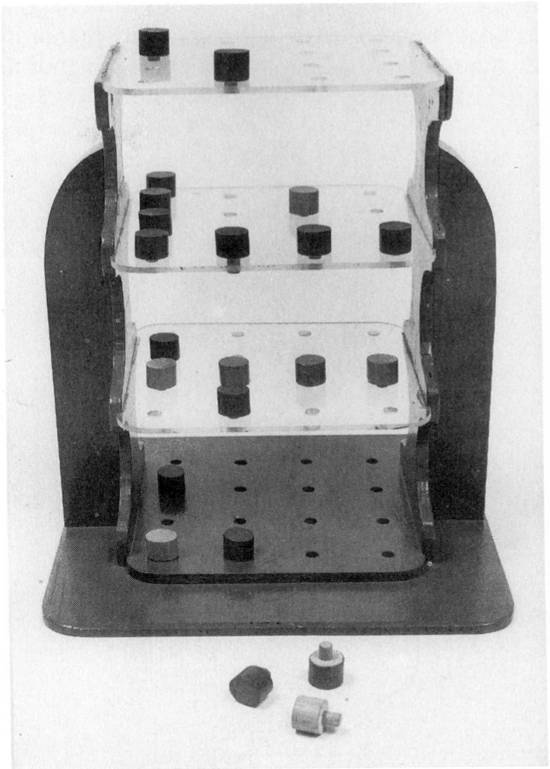

pronation and supination. The aim of the activity is to pass a washer along the wire from one end to the other. They can be graded for difficulty according to the amount and complexity of twists in the wire (Fig. 6.8). Methods to increase the difficulty value include increasing or decreasing the size of the washer bore, and changing the type of washer used (a soft one will be infinitely more difficult than a metal one).

To achieve shoulder movement, the patient must keep his elbow in extension (if necessary within a plastazote cylinder).

**Fig. 6.8** Three dimensional noughts and crosses.

### THE MARBLE GAME

This is a simple activity designed to promote both wrist and finger extension in addition to wrist flexion. The marbles are placed in a drawer, which is con-

tained within the main body of the game. The forearm is rested along the gutter and strapped into place with the two retaining straps. The patient therefore has to flex the wrist to collect a marble, then place this marble through a hole in the upright

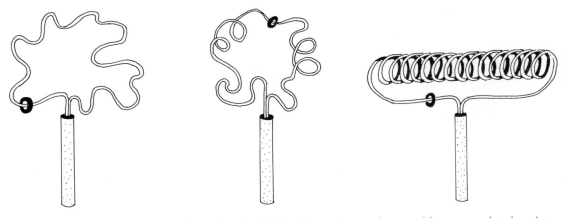

**Fig. 6.9** Coathanger-wire 'twisters' graded in order of difficulty. The washer must be passed from one end to the other.

section. In performing this act, maximum wrist and finger extension are achieved. The higher the hole that the marble is put through, the higher the score. This score is useful not only for the setting of targets but also to serve as a record of progress (Fig. 6.10).

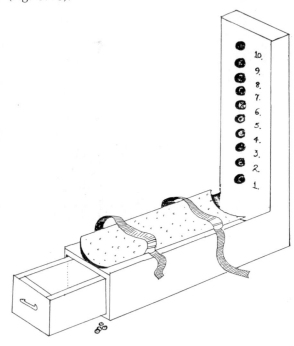

**Fig. 6.10** The marble game entails picking up a marble from the box underneath and placing it in as high a hole in the column as possible.

## THE LENTIL GAME

This is a very useful warming up activity, providing sensory stimulation with multiple unresisted finger and wrist movements. The patient places his hand firstly into water, and secondly palm down onto a flat surface generously covered with lentils. Having removed the hand from the lentils, the patient must attempt to dislodge those that are adhering to the palm and fingers, without using the other hand. Shaking of the hand is not allowed.

To increase the difficulty value:
(i) Wet the hand in tepid or warm water (this increases the vacuum created and makes the lentils harder to dislodge).
(ii) Increase the amount of times the activity is performed.

To decrease the difficulty value:
—Substitute another pulse for the lentils (for example rice).

## ELASTIC BOXES ACTIVITY

This is an activity that promotes active abduction and passive adduction of the fingers. The patient has to stretch rubber bands over pins or nails, which have been hammered into a board. If the activity is to be competitive, the patient must (by taking alternative turns with his opponent) attempt to make as many boxes as possible, stretching the band over a minimum of four nails. Failure to make a box, or loss of the band will not count as a score.

To increase the difficulty value:
(i) Increase the resistance of the bands.
(ii) Space the pins or nails further apart.
(iii) Progressively increase the number of nails that the patient must stretch the band around.

## SENSORY ACTIVITIES

Any hand activity will provide varying degrees of sensory stimulation, although assessment and treatment ones should not overlap lest a learning bias results. Activities such as finding objects hidden in rice, dried peas or polystyrene granules are useful not only for sensory input, but also for desensitising areas, such as amputation stumps.

Hand games may easily be adapted by the introduction of different textures, for example textured dominoes.

## CONCLUSION

Games are a useful adjunct to hand therapy, but like specific exercise, may quickly become repetitive for the patient undergoing a prolonged period of intensive treatment. Morale is of major importance in the continuing motivation of the hand patient, and it is therefore of value to include some functional tasks. In the absence of an occupational therapy department, a measure of compromise may be offered by the addition of clerical activities

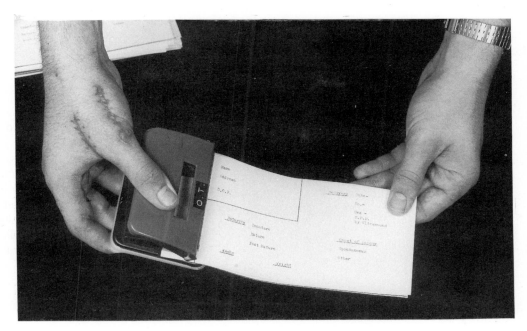

**Fig. 6.11** Clerical activities can offer a variety of useful hand functions.

to the treatment programme. Such activities could include collating, stapling, filing, typing and computer operating. Hospital departments who deal in educational handouts may be only too willing to let hand patients collate packages. Similarly, the sorting, punching (Fig. 6.11) and stapling of handouts for courses may also be of use to the secretarial department, as may the simple folding and packing of new hospital notes folders.

Occupational therapy by merit of its ability to offer general or specific functional activities, well complements the specific exercises and treatments of physiotherapy. It provides the necessary additional stimulus through graded activity, in the areas of activities of daily living or in light and heavy workshops, where specific tasks are well balanced with work assessment, job simulation and retraining activities. It is thus that occupational therapy can employ different aspects of motivation to achieve similar objectives to the physiotherapist, whilst both must vitally work together towards the common goal of good hand rehabilitation.

## ACKNOWLEDGEMENTS

I would like to extend my grateful thanks to Miss K.M. Fielding (District Head Occupational Therapist) and Mrs J.I. Kerley (Research Physiotherapist) for advice and help concerning the text; to Dr I.D. Swain for use of his department's word processing facility; and to the Wessex Rehabilitation Association for assistance with typing.

## FURTHER READING

Jones M, Jay P 1977 An approach to Occupational therapy, 3rd edn. Butterworths, London
Trombly C A, Scott A D 1983 Occupational therapy for physical dysfunction, 2nd edn. Williams & Wilkins, Baltimore
Turner A 1987 The practice of Occupational therapy—an introduction to the treatment of physical dysfunction, 2nd edn. Churchill Livingstone, Edinburgh

# Index

$44.05